OXFORD MEDICAL PUBLICATIONS

The Causes of Cancer

The Causes of Cancer

Quantitative Estimates of
Avoidable Risks of Cancer in the
United States Today

Richard Doll, F.R.S.
and
Richard Peto

OXFORD · NEW YORK
OXFORD UNIVERSITY PRESS

Oxford University Press, Walton Street, Oxford OX2 6DP

Oxford New York Toronto
Delhi Bombay Calcutta Madras Karachi
Petaling Jaya Singapore Hong Kong Tokyo
Nairobi Dar es Salaam Cape Town
Melbourne Auckland
and associated companies in
Beirut Berlin Ibadan Nicosia

Oxford is a trade mark of Oxford University Press

Published in the United States of America
by Oxford University Press, New York

First published in the Journal of the National Cancer
Institute, Volume 66, June 1981, and published by Oxford
University Press by kind permission of the Editor in Chief, 1981
Reprinted 1983 (with corrections), 1984, 1986

Library of Congress Cataloging in Publication Data

Doll, Richard, Sir.
The causes of cancer. (Oxford medical publications)
Bibliography: p.   includes index.
1. Carcinogenesis. 2. Cancer—United States—
Prevention. 3. Epidemiology. I. Peto, Richard,
1943– . II. Title [DNLM: I. Neoplasms—
Etiology. 2. Neoplasms—Prevention and control.
QZ 202 D665c]
RC268.5.D64   616.99'4071   81–11255   AACR2
ISBN 0–19–261359–6 (pbk.)

Printed in Great Britain
at the University Printing House, Oxford
by David Stanford
Printer to the University

PREFACE

The percentage of today's fatal cancers that might, by suitable preventive measures, have been avoided is subject to some dispute. Indeed, the percentage avoidable by certain particular categories of preventive measure is subject to such vigorous dispute that the non-specialist (to whom the present review is addressed) may wonder whether research has yet discovered any solid facts at all about the avoidance of human cancer.

The truth seems to be that there is quite good evidence that cancer is largely an avoidable (although not necessarily a modern) disease, but, with some important exceptions, frustratingly poor evidence as to exactly what are the really important ways of avoiding a reasonable percentage of today's cancers. Perhaps because of this uncertainty, the number of different areas of current research into hypothetical ways of avoiding cancer is enormous. As a convenient framework in which to seek an overview of them all, we have divided the various hypothetical ways of increasing or decreasing cancer onset rates into a dozen groups, and for each such group we have attempted to review what is known about the percentage of current U.S. cancer deaths that might thereby be avoidable.

In some groups (e.g., smoking habits) the quantitative knowledge already available is quite reliable, whereas in others (e.g., dietary habits) it is not, and we have had to fall back on reviewing various current lines of research whose eventual outcome is still unknown. The "percentages" (of current cancer mortality thus avoidable) that we eventually cite for the separate groups are therefore not really comparable with each other. Some are fairly precisely known, whereas others are much less so. More importantly, some relate to quite specific preventive measures on which action would, at least in principle, be possible on present knowledge alone, whereas others relate to preventive measures (e.g., modification of dietary factors) where the changes that would be beneficial have not yet been reliably characterized. Moreover, even if two particular agents (e.g., asbestos and sunlight) happen to account for a similar percentage of all cancer deaths, that which is the more easily controlled is obviously of greater public health significance. Despite all these drawbacks, the "percentages" that we have attributed to each way or group of ways of avoiding cancer remain for us a useful summary of certain facts, and the estimation of those "percentages" remains a convenient way of structuring our review of the quantitative information that is already available or is emerging about the determinants of human cancer.

Our report consists of a review of the evidence that cancer is largely an avoidable disease, a review of recent upward or downward trends in the onset rates of various types of cancer, a review of our reasons for preferring an epidemiological rather than a laboratory-based approach to the quantitative attribution of human risk, and then a dozen separate sections, one on each of the possible ways or groups of ways of avoiding cancer. The final section then summarizes and brings together our principal conclusions. We have relegated most of our detailed discussions of trends and certain other matters to appendixes, for although these details might be of interest to the specialist our principal aim has been to explain matters to interested non-specialists. Of course some isolated pockets of detail remain in the text, but we have used paragraph subheadings fairly liberally throughout in the hope that wherever any reader feels the amount of detail excessive a few pages can be skipped without losing the general sense of our argument.

Finally, following Russell (1946), a few words of apology and explanation are called for, chiefly addressed to the specialists on the various subjects we touch on. Most of these subjects, with the possible exception of tobacco, are better known to some others than to us. If reports covering a wide field are to be written at all it is inevitable, since we are not immortal, that those who write them should spend less time on any one part than can be spent by someone who concentrates on a single subject. Some, whose scholarly austerity is unbending, will conclude that reports covering a wide field should not be written at all, or, if written, should consist of chapters by a multitude of authors. There is, however, something lost when many authors cooperate. If any balance is to be achieved between the findings in laboratory experiments and the distribution of disease that actually occurs in the population as a whole, and if the major and minor causes of death are to be seen in proper perspective, then the various aspects should be synthesized in a consistent way, which would have increased in difficulty exponentially with the number of authors.

This article was commissioned as a report to the Office of Technology Assessment, U.S. Congress, to provide background material for their assessment of "Technologies for Determining Cancer Risks From the Environment" (OTA, 1981).

Acknowledgments

First and foremost, we wish to thank Mrs. Virginia Godwin for her assistance in preparing this report, and we are particularly indebted to Eugene Rogot, of the National Heart, Lung, and Blood Institute, for making available to us the data from the study of a quarter of a million U.S. veterans. Robert Fensterheim abstracted the cancer mortality data from 1933–78 from Government publications, and a tape of these data is available from R. Peto. The staff of the Populations Division of the Bureau of the Census provided corrected U.S. population estimates from 1950, Irene Stratton and Richard Gray analyzed the mortality data, and Cathy Harwood drew the figures. The Surveillance, Epidemiology, and End Results section of the Biometry Branch of the National Cancer Institute and the New York and Connecticut tumor registries kindly provided us with access to cancer incidence data. Finally, we wish to thank the dozens of known or anonymous scientists who, through us or through the Office of Technology Assessment, scrutinized and offered helpful criticism of previous versions of this report. Dr. Michael Gough, as OTA project officer, encouraged us throughout this project.

ABBREVIATIONS USED: ACS = American Cancer Society; AF2 = 2-(2-furyl)-3-(5-nitro-2-furyl)acrylamide; CPEAP = Committee on Prototype Explicit Analyses for Pesticides; DAB = p-dimethylaminoazobenzene; DES = diethylstilbestrol; DMBA = 7,12-dimethylbenz[a]anthracene; EPA = Environmental Protection Agency; GESAMP = Group of Experts on the Scientific Aspects of Marine Pollution; IARC = International Agency for Research on Cancer; ICD = International Classification of Diseases; NAS = National Academy of Sciences; NCI = National Cancer Institute; NIOSH = National Institute of Occupational Safety and Health; NIEHS = National Institute of Environmental Health Sciences; OSHA = Occupational Safety and Health Administration; PVC = polyvinyl chloride; SEER = Surveillance, Epidemiology, and End Results program of NCI; SNCS = Second National Cancer Survey; TNCS = Third National Cancer Survey; TSSC = Toxic Substances Strategy Committee; WHO = World Health Organization.

TABLE OF CONTENTS

ABSTRACT—Evidence that the various common types of cancer are largely avoidable diseases is reviewed. Life-style and other environmental factors are divided into a dozen categories, and for each category the evidence relating those particular factors to cancer onset rates is summarized. Where possible, an estimate is made of the percentage of current U.S. cancer mortality that might have been caused or avoided by that category of factors. These estimates are based chiefly on evidence from epidemiology, as the available evidence from animal and other laboratory studies cannot provide reliable human risk assessments. By far the largest reliably known percentage is the 30% of current U.S. cancer deaths that are due to tobacco, although it is possible that some nutritional factor(s) may eventually be found to be of comparable importance. The percentage of U.S. cancer deaths that are due to tobacco is still increasing, and must be expected to continue to increase for some years yet due to the delayed effects of the adoption of cigarettes in earlier decades.

Trends in mortality and in onset rates for many separate types of cancer are studied in detail in appendixes to this paper. Biases in the available data on registration of new cases produce apparent trends in cancer incidence which are spurious. Biases also produce spurious trends in cancer death certification rates, especially among old people. In (and before) middle age, where the biases are smaller, there appear to be a few real increases and a few real decreases in mortality from some particular types of cancer, but there is no evidence of any generalized increase other than that due to tobacco. Moderate increases or decreases due to some new agent(s) or habit(s) might of course be overlooked in such large-scale analyses. But, such analyses do suggest that, apart from cancer of the respiratory tract, the types of cancer that are currently common are not peculiarly modern diseases and are likely to depend chiefly on some long-established factor(s). (A prospective study utilizing both questionnaires and stored blood and other biological materials might help elucidate these factors.)

The proportion of current U.S. cancer deaths attributed to occupational factors is provisionally estimated as 4% (lung cancer being the major contributor to this). This is far smaller than has recently been suggested by various U.S. Government agencies. The matter could be resolved directly by a "case–control" study of lung cancer two or three times larger than the recently completed U.S. National Bladder Cancer Study but similar to it in methodology and unit costs; there are also other reasons for such a study.

A fuller summary of conclusions and recommendations comprises the final section of this report.—JNCI 1981; 66:1191–1308.

1. DEFINITION OF AVOIDABILITY OF CANCER

The various human cancers are diseases in which one of the many cells of which the human body is composed is altered in such a way that it inappropriately replicates itself again and again, producing millions of similarly affected self-replicating descendant cells, some of which may spread to other parts of the body and eventually overwhelm it.[1] Some cancers are easily curable; whereas others are almost always completely incurable by the time they are diagnosed, depending largely on the organ of the body (lung, larynx, large intestine, etc.) in which the first altered cell originated. The symptoms produced and the approach to treatment also vary with the site of origin, so that it has been customary for doctors to regard tumors originating from different organs as different diseases. Gradually, it has come to be realized that agents or habits which greatly increase or decrease the likelihood of one particular type of cancer arising (in humans or experimental animals) may have little effect on most other types of cancer, so that the prevention of each type also must be considered separately. This realization reinforces the need to consider cancers of different organs as largely independent diseases, just as we have to consider separately different infectious diseases such as syphilis, smallpox, and tuberculosis. When we consider them separately, we see at once that although there are several dozen different organs from which tumors may arise, cancers of three organs (lung, breast, and large intestine) are at present of outstanding importance as they currently account for half the U.S. cancer deaths (table 1). A substantial reduction in any of these three cancers, particularly lung cancer, would materially reduce total U.S. cancer death rates, whereas such reductions in any other type of cancer would have relatively little effect.

That the common fatal cancers occur in large part as a result of life-style and other environmental factors and are in principle preventable was recognized by an expert committee of the WHO in 1964. The committee, which had been appointed to consider how existing knowledge could be applied to prevent cancer, began its report (WHO, 1964) by stating that:

The potential scope of cancer prevention is limited by the proportion of human cancers in which extrinsic factors are responsible. These [factors] include all environmental carcinogens (whether identified or not) as well as 'modifying factors' that favour neoplasia of apparently intrinsic origin (e.g., hormonal imbalances, dietary deficiencies and metabolic defects). The categories of cancer that are thus influenced, directly or indirectly, by extrinsic factors include many tumours of the skin and mouth, the respiratory,

TABLE 1.—*Numbers of deaths certified as being due to various types of tumor: United States, 1978*

Type of tumor	No. of deaths	Percent of all deaths from tumors	
Cancer of the			
Lung[a]	95,086	24	
Large bowel (colon and rectum)	53,269	13	46
Breast	34,609	9	
Prostate	21,674	5	
Pancreas	20,777	5	46
Stomach	14,452	4	
29 other types or categories,[b] each contributing less than 3% of deaths	128,705	32	
Other or unspecified tumors[c]	33,383	8	
Total, all tumors	401,955	100	

[a] The annual number of lung cancer deaths is changing rapidly and will probably be ≈105,000 by 1981. If it is, cancers of the lung, breast, and large intestine will account for just over half of all deaths from tumors where the site of origin of the tumor was specified on the death certificate (*see* footnote *c*).
[b] Including all leukemias as one category. (A detailed breakdown by sex and site is available in tables 17–19, pp. 1243–1244.)
[c] Comprising 4,963 deaths attributed to tumors of benign or unspecified histology, and 28,420 deaths attributed to cancer for which the site of origin was not specified; at least half of the latter probably originated from the six commonest sites.

gastrointestinal and urinary tracts, hormone dependent organs (such as the breast, thyroid and uterus), haematopoietic and lymphopoietic systems, which, collectively, account for more than three-quarters of human cancers. It would seem, therefore, that the majority of human cancer is potentially preventible.

Many individuals had already expressed this belief previously, and the committee's report merely served to indicate that a consensus among most cancer research workers had been achieved. In the years since that report was published, advances in knowledge have consolidated these opinions and few if any competent research workers now question its main conclusion. Individuals, indeed, have gone further and have substituted figures of 80 or even 90% as the proportion of potentially preventable cancers in place of the 1964 committee's cautious estimate of "the majority."

Unfortunately, the phrase "extrinsic factors" (or the phrase "environmental factors," which is often substituted for it) has been misinterpreted by many people to mean only "man-made chemicals," which was certainly not the intent of the WHO committee. The committee included, in addition to man-made or natural carcinogens, viral infections, nutritional deficiencies or excesses, reproductive activities, and a variety of other factors determined wholly or partly by personal behavior. To avoid similar misunderstandings, we shall refer throughout this report to the percentages of cancers that "might be avoidable" in various ways, rather than to the percentages that are due to various "extrinsic" or "environmental" factors, and have used the term "avoidable" in our title. We have had in mind throughout our report the avoidance of cancer only by

---

[1] "Tumor" and "neoplasm" have similar meanings, but strictly the word "cancer" relates only to invasive solid tumors of certain tissues. However, most fatal tumors are "cancers" and we shall sometimes use this familiar term loosely to include both solid and diffuse malignant neoplasms plus sometimes even the fatal benign tumors as well.

means that might conceivably be socially acceptable, either now or in some plausible social atmosphere in the reasonably near future. (Potentially acceptable measures might, for example, include a continuation of the current decrease in cigarette smoking or tar yields, which would reduce the risk of lung cancer, but would not include a first pregnancy for most females by 15 years of age, though this would reduce the risk of breast cancer.) Even with this restriction, however, two ambiguities remain in what is meant by the "avoidability" of cancer.

First, by the year 2100 advances in basic research in biology may permit prevention of cancer by means now utterly unforeseen. No useful estimate of the likelihood of such progress can be made, and we have therefore tried to restrict our attention chiefly to the avoidability of cancer by means whose effects on cancer risks are already reasonably certain or by means that might well be devised over the next decade or two rather than in the indefinite future. For this we have not assumed that the mechanisms underlying such means are known or will be known in the near future, but chiefly that it should be possible to identify those things which different groups of people already do, or have done to them, that account for the marked differences in cancer risk between or within communities and that this identification will in many instances lead to preventive strategies which are based either directly or indirectly on the ways in which some people already live and are therefore reasonably practical.

A second, more trivial, ambiguity in what we mean by the "avoidability" of cancer arises simply because everybody is bound to die sooner or later. (If there are about two million births per year in the United States, there are in the long run also bound to be about two million deaths per year.) If exactly half the cancer deaths that now occur were somehow magically prevented and nothing else changed, those people who would have died of cancer might live on for a further 5, 10, 20, or 30 more years (the average being 10 or 15 extra years), but they must eventually die of something and that something would for some of them be a second cancer. Even so, we would still describe such a change as a *halving* of the cancer rate. To take an opposite example, if every cause of death other than cancer were suddenly abolished then of course everyone would eventually die of cancer, although it might be misleading to describe such a change in terms of an increase in either the risk of cancer or the average age at death from cancer, especially if one were interested in the causes of cancer. The usual means of avoiding such absurdities is to avoid basing inferences on the percentage of people who "will eventually" die of cancer, on "crude" cancer rates, or on "the mean age at death from cancer." Instead, it is usual to restrict attention to "age-specific" or "age-standardized" cancer rates (*see* appendixes A and B). When we speak of the avoidance of a certain percentage of cancer, we therefore have in mind a reduction by that percentage in the age-standardized rates. (This may sound complicated,

but it is merely the arithmetic equivalent of not advising people that the most reliable way of avoiding cancer is to commit suicide.)

In summary, the aim of our report is to review the established evidence and current research relating to each of several different possible ways or groups of ways of avoiding cancer and to estimate the percentage reduction in today's age-standardized U.S. cancer death rates that they might confer, now or in the medium-term future.

2. EVIDENCE FOR THE AVOIDABILITY OF CANCER

The evidence that much human cancer is avoidable can be summarized under four heads: differences in the incidence of cancer among different settled communities, differences between migrants from a community and those who remain behind, variations with time in the incidence of cancer within particular communities, and the actual identification of many specific causes or preventive factors. Genetic factors and age also affect cancer onset rates, of course, but this does not affect the conclusion that much human cancer is avoidable.

2.1 Differences in Incidence Between Communities

Evidence of differences in the incidence[2] of particular types of cancer between different parts of the world has accumulated slowly over the past 50 years. At first the only quantitative data available referred to mortality[2] rates in particular areas or, even more crudely, to the proportion of patients admitted to hospital suffering from different diseases. Such data were grossly affected by the age distribution of the population, the efficacy of treatment, and the frequency of other diseases. But even then data were sufficient to show that the incidence of some cancers among people of a given age in different parts of the world must vary by at least ten and possibly by a hundredfold. More recently, this evidence has been reinforced by the results of special surveys or by the establishment of registries in which records are consistently sought of all cases of cancer diagnosed in a defined population over a long period. Registry data also need care in interpretation owing to trends with time, or differences between different parts of the world, in the provision of medical services and in the extent to which they are used (especially by old people, among whom a large proportion of fatal cancers may never be diagnosed at all). Reasonably reliable comparisons between different areas are obtained only if comparisons are limited to men and women in middle life (or earlier, for some specific types of cancer), when a sufficient number of cases can be anticipated for onset rates to be reliably estimated and yet efforts at diagnosis are still likely to be

---

[2] Definition: The *incidence* (rate) depends on the total number of new cases of cancer (per year), while the *mortality* (rate), also called the death rate, ignores non-fatal cases.

thorough. The International Union Against Cancer (1970) and IARC (1976) have recommended that, for the cancers of adult life, attention be chiefly directed to the risks in the truncated age range of 35-64 years (and many artifacts of interpretation of trends in U.S. cancer data might be avoided if this simple precaution were generally adopted).

Table 2 shows for 19 common types of cancer their range of variation among those cancer registries that have produced data sufficiently reliable to be published for the purposes of international comparison by the IARC (1976) and the International Union Against Cancer (1966 and 1970). Types of cancer have been included if they are common enough somewhere to affect more than 1% of men (or women) by 75 years of age in the absence of other causes of death, and ranges of variation are shown for standardized incidence rates between 35 and 64 years of age.[3]

The range of variation (table 2) is never less than sixfold and is commonly much more. Some of this variation may be artifactual, due to different standards of medical service, case registration, and population enumeration, despite the care taken to exclude unreliable data; but in many cases the true ranges will be

greater. First, large gaps remain in the cancer map of the world, and some extreme figures may have been overlooked because no accurate surveys have been practicable in the least developed areas, these being just the areas that are likely to provide the biggest contrasts (both high and low) with Western society. Second, the rates cited in table 2 refer to cancers of whole organs, and in one particular organ such as the stomach, liver, or skin there may be many different types of cells that are affected differently by different carcinogens or protective factors; for example, in the skin the few cancers arising from the cells that are responsible for the manufacture of the dark pigment melanin in blacks or in suntanned whites are called "melanomas," and differ greatly in etiology and prognosis from the many "non-melanoma skin cancers." Third, various anatomic parts of one single organ such as the colon or skin may be affected differently by different factors; for example, cancers of the skin have different principal causes in the populations where they are common depending on whether they chiefly appear on the face, abdomen, forearm, or legs. Finally, although cancers of the skin are so common in certain parts of the world that they outnumber all other cancers, most are so easily cured that they engender little medical interest and are commonly not reported to, or in some cases sought by, even some of the best cancer registries. For these reasons and because the extremes of variation in skin cancer incidence between different communities are affected by skin color as well as by the means of avoidance which chiefly interest us, skin cancers (other than melanomas) are perhaps of less interest than any other type of cancer in table 2.

[3] The incidence of most types of cancer increases with age so rapidly that it may be misleading to compare disease onset rates among people in one part of the world with those of people elsewhere if the proportions of people of different ages in the populations being compared are not the same. This particular difficulty may be circumvented by the use of age-standardized incidence rates (*see* appendix A), and the rates in table 2 are standardized as recommended by the IARC (1976).

TABLE 2.—*Range of incidence rates for common cancers among males (and for certain cancers among females)*

Site of origin of cancer	High incidence area	Sex	Cumulative incidence,[a] % in high incidence area	Ratio of highest rate to lowest rate[b]	Low incidence area
Skin (chiefly non-melanoma)	Australia, Queensland	♂	>20	>200	India, Bombay
Esophagus	Iran, northeast section	♂	20	300	Nigeria
Lung and bronchus	England	♂	11	35	Nigeria
Stomach	Japan	♂	11	25	Uganda
Cervix uteri	Colombia	♀	10	15	Israel: Jewish
Prostate	United States: blacks	♂	9	40	Japan
Liver	Mozambique	♂	8	100	England
Breast	Canada, British Columbia	♀	7	7	Israel: non-Jewish
Colon	United States, Connecticut	♂	3	10	Nigeria
Corpus uteri	United States, California	♀	3	30	Japan
Buccal cavity	India, Bombay	♂	2	25	Denmark
Rectum	Denmark	♂	2	20	Nigeria
Bladder	United States, Connecticut	♂	2	6	Japan
Ovary	Denmark	♀	2	6	Japan
Nasopharynx	Singapore: Chinese	♂	2	40	England
Pancreas	New Zealand: Maori	♂	2	8	India, Bombay
Larynx	Brazil, São Paulo	♂	2	10	Japan
Pharynx	India, Bombay	♂	2	20	Denmark
Penis	Parts of Uganda	♂	1	300	Israel: Jewish

[a] By age 75 yr, in the absence of other causes of death.
[b] At ages 35-64 yr, standardized for age as in IARC (1976). At these ages, even the data from cancer registries in poor countries are likely to be reasonably reliable (although at older ages serious underreporting may affect the data).

Variation in incidence is not, of course, limited to the types of cancer that are common enough somewhere in the world to have been included in table 2. For example, Burkitt's lymphoma has nowhere been found in over 0.1% of the population, but even so is 100 times less common in North America than in the West Nile district of Uganda. Also, Kaposi's sarcoma, which is extremely rare in most of the world, is so common in parts of Central Africa that it accounted for more than 10% of all tumors seen in the (mostly young) males in one hospital (Cook and Burkitt, 1971). Some few rather rare types of cancer, such as the nephroblastoma of childhood, may perhaps eventually be shown to occur with approximately the same frequency in all communities; but no common types of cancer will be found to do so. In the absence of other causes of death, cancer of the breast would affect about 6% of U.S. women before the age of 75 years as against only 1% of non-Jewish Israeli women, and it is possible that an even lower percentage would be affected in certain other populations where reliable cancer registries do not yet exist. With breast cancer as the only possible exception, for each type of cancer a population exists where the cumulative incidence by the age of 75 years is well under 1%. In other words, every type of cancer that is common in one district is rare somewhere else.

Most of the figures in table 2 refer to the incidence of cancer in different communities defined by the area in which they live. Communities can, however, be defined in other ways and no matter how they are defined (whether by ethnic origin, religion, or economic status) similar or sometimes even greater differences will be found. Of particular interest are some of the differences that have been observed in the United States between members of different religious groups.[4] For example, in comparison with members of other religious groups living in the same States, the Mormons of Utah and the Seventh-day Adventists and Mormons of California experience low incidence rates for cancers of the respiratory, gastrointestinal, and genital systems.

Of course, it is unlikely that any one single community will by chance have the highest rates in the world for every single type of cancer, just as it is unlikely that any one single community will by chance have the lowest rates in the world for every single type of cancer. Consequently, when we consider total cancer rates, which are obtained by adding the rates for each separate type of cancer, in various communities we find less extreme variation (only threefold) between communities around the world than was found for many separate single types of cancer. However, there is if anything still *more* variation in these total cancer incidence rates than would have been expected if for each community the rates for the separate single types of cancer had been picked at random from the corresponding rates around the world for single types of cancer (Peto J: Unpublished calculations based on IARC, 1976). Consequently, the relative constancy of total cancer incidence rates around the world does not suggest that if one cancer is prevented another will tend to replace it;[5] it merely shows that if many things are added up, irregularities will tend to be averaged out.

Apart from cancer of the skin, the risk of which is much greater for whites than for blacks (and possibly also apart from the consistent lack among people of Chinese or Japanese descent of certain lymphoproliferative conditions) it does not seem likely that most of the large differences in cancer onset rates between communities could be chiefly due to genetic factors (*see* section 2.5), and such factors certainly cannot explain the differences observed on migration or with the passage of time that are described in the following sections.

2.2 Changes in Incidence on Migration

Evidence of a change in the incidence of cancer in a migrant group (from that in the homeland they have left toward that of their new country of residence) provides good evidence of the importance of life-style or other environmental factors in the production of the disease. That such changes have occurred and are occurring is beyond reasonable doubt, but strictly controlled quantitative evidence comparing incidence rates in the three populations (original country, migrant group, and new country) is hard to come by. Black Americans, for example, experience cancer incidence rates that are generally much more like those of white Americans than like those of the black population in West Africa from which they were originally drawn, as is indicated for selected sites[6] in table 3. From the strict scientific point of view, this comparison is unsatisfactory because the ancestors of black Americans would have come from many different parts of (chiefly West) Africa, some of which are likely to have cancer rates somewhat different from those observed in Nigeria. Nevertheless, the contrast is so great that there can be little doubt that new factors were

---

[4] *See*, for example, the papers from the recent workshop on "Cancer and Mortality in Religious Groups": Lyon et al., 1980a; Lyon et al., 1980b; Enstrom, 1980; West et al., 1980; Phillips et al., 1980; Martin et al., 1980; King and Locke, 1980a.

[5] The suggestion that environmental and life-style factors do not usually have much effect on whether or when an individual gets cancer, but merely affect the site at which a (hypothetically) predestined cancer will appear, has recurred from time to time for half a century ever since Cramer (1934) overlooked the fact that the coefficient of variation of total cancer rates must of necessity be less than that of individual cancer rates. It is easily disproved by noting that people exposed to hazards (e.g., carcinogens in industry or cigarette smoke: Doll, 1978) which affect specific types of cancer do not have reduced risks of cancer of any other type. The same is, of course, true among experimental animals.

[6] We omitted data for cancer sites for which the Ibadan rates resemble the U.S. white rates (e.g., esophagus and stomach).

TABLE 3.—*Comparison of cancer incidence rates[a] for Ibadan, Nigeria, and for two populations of blacks and whites in the United States*

Primary site of cancer	Patients' sex[c]	Annual incidence/million people[b]		
		Ibadan, Nigeria, 1960–69	United States[d]	
			Blacks	Whites
Colon	♂	34	349	294
			353	335
Rectum	♂	34	159	217
			248	232
Liver	♂	272	67	39
			86	32
Pancreas	♂	55	200	126
			250	122
Larynx	♂	37	236	141
			149	141
Lung	♂	27	1,546	983
			1,517	979
Prostate	♂	134	724	318
			577	232
Breast	♀	337	1,268	1,828
			1,105	1,472
Cervix uteri	♀	559	507	249
			631	302
Corpus uteri	♀	42	235	695
			208	441
Lymphosarcoma[e] at ages <15 yr	♂	133	10	4
			5	3

[a] From IARC (1976).
[b] Ages 35–64 yr, standardized for age as in IARC (1976).
[c] For brevity, wherever possible only the male rates have been presented, and sites for which the rates among U S whites resemble those in the country of origin of the non-white migrants have been omitted.
[d] For each type of cancer, upper entry shows incidence in San Francisco Bay area, 1969–73; lower entry shows incidence in Detroit, 1969–71.
[e] Including Burkitt's lymphoma. The cited rates are the average of the age-specific rates at ages 0–4, 5–9 and 10–14 yr.

introduced with migration. These, it would appear, are not chiefly the result of genetic dilution by interbreeding, for at most major sites the differences between black and white Americans in defined areas seem largely independent of the degree of admixture of white-derived genes among the blacks in those areas (Petrakis, 1971).

A similar comparison can be made between the Japanese and Caucasian residents in Hawaii and the Japanese in two particular prefectures of Japan (table 4). The close approximation of the rates in the two prefectures gives some justification for believing that they may be typical of the areas from which the Japanese migrants to Hawaii (or their ancestors) originated, although the migrants will have come from other parts of Japan as well. For every type of cancer except cancer of the lung, the rates for the migrants are more like those for the Caucasian residents than for those in Japan.

Other groups for which data are available include Indians who went to Fiji and South Africa (and lost their high risk of developing oral cancer), Britons who went to Fiji (and acquired a high risk of skin cancer), and Central Europeans who went to North America and Australia. Data for some of these groups were reviewed in 1969, under the auspices of the International Agency for Research on Cancer (Haenszel, 1970; Kmet, 1970), and recent data on cancer patterns in different ethnic groups within the United States were reviewed in 1980 under the auspices of the National Cancer Institute (Kolonel, 1980; King and Locke, 1980b; Locke and King, 1980; Lanier et al., 1980).

2.3 Changes in Incidence Over Time

Changes in the incidence of particular types of cancer with the passage of time provide conclusive evidence that extrinsic factors affect those types of cancer. Such changes are, however, notoriously difficult to estimate reliably, chiefly because it is difficult to compare the efficiency of case finding at different periods and partly because few incidence data have been collected for a sufficiently long time, so that we have to compare mortality rates, which record only fatal cases and thus may be influenced by changes in treatment. There are no uniform rules for deciding which of the many apparent changes in cancer incidence are real. Each set of incidence data and each type of cancer must be assessed individually. It is relatively easy to be sure about changes in the incidence of cancer of the esophagus, because the disease can be diagnosed without complex investigations and its oc-

TABLE 4.—*Comparison of cancer incidence rates[a] in Japan and for Japanese and Caucasians in Hawaii*

Primary site of cancer	Patients' sex[c]	Annual incidence/million people[b]		
		Japan[d]	Hawaii, 1968–72	
			Japanese	Caucasians
Esophagus	♂	150	46	75
		112		
Stomach	♂	1,331	397	217
		1,291		
Colon	♂	78	371	368
		87		
Rectum	♂	95	297	204
		90		
Lung	♂	237	379	962
		299		
Prostate	♂	14	154	343
		13		
Breast	♀	335	1,221	1,869
		295		
Cervix uteri	♀	329	149	243
		398		
Corpus uteri	♀	32	407	714
		20		
Ovary	♀	51	160	274
		55		

[a] From IARC (1976).
[b] Ages 35–64 yr, standardized for age as in IARC (1976).
[c] Male only, wherever possible; sites selected as in table 3.
[d] For each type of cancer, upper entry shows incidence in Miyagi prefecture, 1968–71; lower entry shows incidence in Osaka prefecture, 1970–71.

currence is nearly always recorded, at least in middle age, for it is nearly always fatal. It is much more difficult to be sure about changes in the incidence of many other types of cancer. The common basal cell carcinomas of the skin, for example, are also easy to diagnose but are often not registered at all, as they seldom cause death and may be treated effectively outside the hospital. What appears to be a change in incidence may, therefore, be a change only in the completeness of registration. Cancer of the pancreas, by contrast, is almost always fatal but is easily misdiagnosed, perhaps as cancer of some other organ, unless it is specially looked for. What appears to be an increased incidence may, therefore, be wholly or partly due to improvements in diagnosis, in the availability of medical services, or (as for all other types of cancer) in the readiness of physicians to inform cancer registries of any cancers they find. Such changes are particularly likely to affect the cancer incidence rates recorded for people over 65 years of age, as many terminally ill old people used not to be intensively investigated (sometimes, it must be admitted, to their advantage).

As most cancers are commoner among the old than among the young, these spurious changes in old age are liable to distort overall rates quite considerably and (if attention is not restricted to people under 65 years of age) may conceal a stable or even a decreasing incidence at younger ages at which cancer has been reasonably well diagnosed for several decades. Despite these difficulties, some changes during periods when no large improvements in relevant diagnostic technology were introduced have been so gross that there can be no doubt about their reality. These changes include the increase in esophageal cancer in the black population of South Africa, the continued increase in lung cancer throughout most of the world, the increase in mesothelioma of the pleura in males in industrialized countries, and the decrease in cancer of the tongue in Britain and in cancers of the cervix uteri and stomach throughout Western Europe and North America. Worldwide changes in the mortality attributed to cancers of the lung and stomach in the last 25 years are given in table 5. Detailed U.S. data for these and many other types of cancer are discussed in section 4.1 and in appendixes C, D, and E.

2.4 Identification of Causes

The simplest evidence of the preventability of cancer would be the demonstration by scientific experiment that a particular action actually leads to a reduction in the incidence of the disease. Even where such evidence could in principle have been sought by means of randomized trials, this has not in general been done, and so we often have to be content with the type of strong circumstantial evidence that would be sufficient to obtain a conviction in a court of law. Action, based on such evidence, has in practice often been followed by the desired result—for example, a reduction in the incidence of bladder cancer in the chemical industry has been seen since stopping the manufacture and use

TABLE 5.—*International changes since 1950 in death certification rates for cancers of stomach and lung*

Country	Period	Percent change in mortality[a] from cancer of:	
		Stomach	Lung
Australia	1950–51 to 1975	−53	+146
Austria	1952–53 to 1976	−53	−8
Chile	1950–51 to 1975	−56	+38
Denmark	1952–53 to 1976	−62	+87
England and Wales	1950–51 to 1975	−49	+33
West Germany	1952–53 to 1975	−50	+36
Ireland	1950–51 to 1975	−54	+177
Israel	1950–51 to 1975	−49	+58
Japan	1950–51 to 1976	−37	+408
The Netherlands	1950–51 to 1976	−60	+89
New Zealand	1950–51 to 1975	−54	+137
Norway	1952–53 to 1975	−59	+118
Scotland	1950–51 to 1975	−46	+44
Switzerland	1952–53 to 1976	−64	+72
United States	1950–51 to 1975	−61	+148

[a] Average of ♂ and ♀ rates at ages 35–64 yr, standardized for age as in IARC (1976).

of 2-naphthylamine, while the progressive increase in lung cancer risk that regular cigarette smokers suffer is avoided by people who give up the habit of smoking. Cancer research workers throughout the world have therefore accepted that the type of human evidence that has been obtained, sometimes but by no means invariably (*see* section 4.2) combined with laboratory evidence that some suspect agent is carcinogenic in animals, is strong enough to justify the conclusion that a means of avoiding some cases of human cancer has been identified. There are, of course, many borderline instances where reasonable differences of opinion exist, while even for the well-established causes a few critics can always be found who will argue that causality is not established. A majority of students of the subject are agreed that a few dozen agents or circumstances have already been shown to cause or prevent cancer in humans and that, in a number of other instances, the conditions that give rise to an increased incidence of cancer have been closely defined without a specific agent having yet been identified (IARC Working Group, 1980). These agents and conditions are listed in table 6. Exposure to some agents, it will be noted, has been on only a small scale, as in the case of a drug introduced briefly for the treatment of a rare disease, whereas exposure to others has been intensive and widespread, and hundreds of thousands of cancers have been caused each year. The extent to which these listed agents and conditions are now affecting the incidence of cancer in the United States is discussed in Section 5.

2.5 Role of Genetic Factors, Luck, and Age

Some people of a given age will develop cancer in the near future, and some will not. The determinants of who will and who will not develop cancer are best divided into three categories, not only the usual "na-

TABLE 6.—*Established human carcinogenic agents and circumstances*[a,b]

Agent or circumstance	Exposure[c]			Site of cancer
	Occupational	Medical	Social	
Aflatoxin			+	Liver
Alcoholic drinks			+	Mouth, pharynx, larynx, eosphagus, liver
Alkylating agents:				
Cyclophosphamide		+		Bladder
Melphalan		+		Marrow
Aromatic amines:				
4-Aminodiphenyl	+			Bladder
Benzidine	+			"
2-Naphthylamine	+			"
Arsenic[d]	+	+		Skin, lung
Asbestos	+			Lung, pleura, peritoneum
Benzene	+			Marrow
Bis(chloromethyl) ether	+			Lung
Busulphan		+		Marrow
Cadmium[d]	+			Prostate
Chewing (betel, tobacco, lime)			+	Mouth
Chromium[d]	+			Lung
Chlornaphazine		+		Bladder
Furniture manufacture (hardwood)	+			Nasal sinuses
Immunosuppressive drugs		+		Reticuloendothelial system
Ionizing radiations[e]	+	+		Marrow and probably all other sites
Isopropyl alcohol manufacture	+			Nasal sinuses
Leather goods manufacture	+			Nasal sinuses
Mustard gas	+			Larynx, lung
Nickel[d]	+			Nasal sinuses, lung
Estrogens:				
Unopposed		+		Endometrium
Transplacental (DES)		+		Vagina
Overnutrition (causing obesity)			+	Endometrium, gallbladder
Phenacetin		+		Kidney (pelvis)
Polycyclic hydrocarbons	+	+		Skin, scrotum, lung
Reproductive history:				
Late age at 1st pregnancy			+	Breast
Zero or low parity			+	Ovary
Parasites:				
Schistosoma haematobium			+	Bladder
Chlonorchis sinensis			+	Liver (cholangioma)
Sexual promiscuity			+	Cervix uteri
Steroids:				
Anabolic (oxymetholone)		+		Liver
Contraceptives		+		Liver (hamartoma)
Tobacco smoking			+	Mouth, pharynx, larynx, lung, esophagus, bladder
UV light	+		+	Skin, lip
Vinyl chloride	+			Liver (angiosarcoma)
Virus (hepatitis B)			+	Liver (hepatoma)

[a] Expanded from IARC working group, 1980.

[b] By restricting this table to firmly established causes, we undoubtedly have omitted some of the more important determinants of human cancer. (A few borderline cases might not command uniform agreement; e.g., we have on balance just included cadmium and just excluded beryllium.)

[c] A plus sign indicates that evidence of carcinogenicity was obtained.

[d] Certain compounds or oxidation states only.

[e] For example, from X-rays, thorium, thorotrast, some underground mining, and other occupations.

Note: Occupational exposure to phenoxyacid/chlorophenol herbicides (or their impurities) is a reasonably well established cause of soft tissue sarcomas and perhaps lymphomas.

ture" and "nurture" but also "luck," or the play of chance. "Nature" relates to a person's genetic makeup at conception, and this certainly affects the risk of some types of cancer. For example, other things being equal, a white-skinned person is more likely to develop skin cancer in response to sunlight than is a black-skinned person, while people who have inherited xero-derma pigmentosum, a very rare genetically determined inability to repair the normal effects of sunlight on the skin (Robbins et al., 1974), are likely to develop several skin cancers per person. "Nurture," which is the subject of this whole report, relates to what people do or have done to them (in the womb, in childhood, or in adult life) and is of public interest as a determinant of cancer risk because it is the only thing that can be influenced by personal or political choice.[7]

Finally, "luck" takes care of the remaining differences in outcome that both observation and theory lead us to expect (Peto, 1977b), perhaps by determining the concatenation of events that brings about specific changes in particular molecules in individual cells at particular times. Somewhat similarly, luck involves some of us but not others in traffic accidents. Even among genetically identical laboratory animals kept under conditions that are as closely uniform as possible, some will die of cancer in middle age, while others will live on into old age with no cancer. (Analogously, the fact that some people die of lung cancer at 40 years of age while other people live on in apparently similar circumstances to 80 does not *of itself* provide any suggestion at all as to whether or not there are any genetic factors which affect lung cancer risks, for variation in age at onset of disease would be expected in either case.)

Nature and nurture affect the probability that each individual will develop cancer, and luck then determines exactly which individuals will actually do so. However, although for each single individual the role of luck is enormous, in a population of a hundred thousand or more (e.g., the population covered by one particular cancer registry) the role of luck is smaller, and in determining the annual number of cancers in the whole United States luck has a completely negligible effect, for the larger the population the more the good and bad luck will tend to average out. Consequently, in the comparison of national cancer rates only nature and nurture are important. Much of the evidence outlined above (changes of cancer incidence with migration, changes over the decades within one country, and the identification of particular causes of cancer) points to an important role for "nurture." However, this does not deny an equally important role for "nature." For example, the stomach cancer risks in certain countries differ markedly from each other, and most are decreasing rapidly (table 5), both of which observations point to the relevance of nurture. However, in both high-risk and low-risk countries people whose "ABO" blood group (a factor that is determined purely genetically) is of type "A" have a stomach cancer risk some 20% greater than that of their compatriots of type "O." In this instance, as for skin cancer, nature and nurture seem to multiply each

other's effects. If many other genetic factors are relevant to stomach cancer, then maybe two compatriots chosen at random would be likely to differ quite widely in their genetic susceptibility to the external causes of stomach cancer, although it is still possible that there is much less individual genetic variation than many people suppose.[8] Whether most Americans are of similar susceptibility or whether there is typically wide variation in susceptibility makes little difference to the net effects of changes in nurture on the total number of cases in the nation as a whole and is therefore of little immediate public health relevance. (In either case, if the causes of stomach cancer are halved, then the stomach cancer rates will be roughly halved, as has been happening every 20 years.) Moreover, even if individuals do vary widely in their genetic susceptibility to stomach cancer, this does not suggest that different countries will vary widely in the averages of the genetic susceptibilities of their citizens, for in each such average all the large variations between compatriots will be ironed out. For a few types of internal cancer the differences between countries may be chiefly due to large differences in genetic susceptibility (e.g., the shortfall of chronic lymphocytic leukemia among the Chinese and Japanese or the excess of cancer of the nasopharynx among the southern Chinese), but this seems likely to be the exception rather than the rule. For example, taking the three types of cancer which are currently commonest in the United States (lung, colorectal, and breast cancers), lung cancer was less than half as common a quarter of a century ago, which shows that most cases are avoidable, while for both breast and colorectal cancers there are striking correlations between the rates in particular countries and various aspects of those countries' life-style (e.g., fat consumption; text-fig. 1). It is most implausible that international variations in daily fat consumption are chiefly determined genetically, and if it is accepted that they are not, then the striking correlations between dietary factors and the onset rates of certain types of cancer show that the large international differences in onset rates are not chiefly genetic in origin. [Note that these correlations merely suggest that these cancers are

---

[7] One difficulty of terminology with the distinction between nature and nurture is where to classify a genetically inherited tendency to behave in certain ways (e.g., to overeat or undereat). From a public health point of view it is probably most appropriate to attribute the net results of tendency-plus-behavior to "nurture," since few such compulsions can be so rigid that social factors will not also affect the behavior pattern. Another difficulty in identifying "nurture" as "that which might be avoidable" is that some day selective abortion (or, more speculatively, selective conception) may be possible to avoid the birth of a few babies with a near certainty of death from cancer.

[8] It is sometimes suggested that because a percentage of smokers do not get lung cancer, there must be other causes, or genetic variability. The conclusion may or may not be correct, but the argument for it is bogus. Conversely, it is often argued that because the relatives of patients with a particular type of cancer have only moderate rather than marked excess risks of that type of cancer (although no excess of cancer in general), the amount of simply inherited genetic susceptibility must also be moderate rather than marked. This argument sounds reasonable, but in fact quite marked genetic variation usually leads to surprisingly moderate excess risks in relatives (Peto J, 1980), so this argument too is bogus unless the analysis is of people with two or more relatives affected by one particular type of cancer (and makes due allowance for familial similarities in life-style and environment). At present, the relevance of genetic susceptibility to the common types of cancer remains obscure.

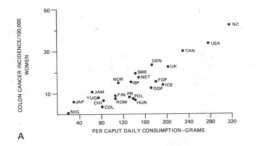

A

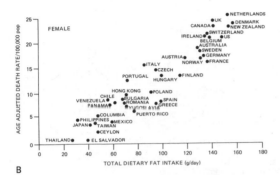

B

TEXT-FIGURE 1.—A) Correlation between colon cancer incidence in various countries and meat consumption (Armstrong and Doll, 1975a; reprinted with permission of *British Journal of Preventive and Social Medicine* and R. Doll). B) Correlation between breast cancer mortality in various countries and fat consumption (Carroll, 1975; reprinted with permission of *Cancer Research* and K. K. Carroll).

These striking age-standardized correlations do not necessarily suggest that either meat or some type of fat are major determinants of either colon or breast cancer, but they do suggest that manipulable determinants of these cancers do exist.

largely avoidable (except perhaps among those few people with the extremely rare genetic conditions of a strong predisposition to colon cancer or to breast cancer at an early age) but do not mean that avoidance of dietary fat would achieve this.]

Turning finally to the role of age itself, it is sometimes suggested that because cancer is ten or a hundred times more likely to arise in the coming year in old people than in young people, aging per se should be thought of as an important determinant of cancer. We rather doubt whether this viewpoint is a scientifically fruitful one (Doll, 1971; Peto et al., 1975), and in any case we are concerned in this report with avoidable causes of cancer, among which we can hardly count old age.

3. PROPORTION OF U.S. CANCERS THAT ARE KNOWN TO BE AVOIDABLE

If the foregoing is accepted as justifying the belief that much human cancer is avoidable, then a crude estimate of the proportion of cases that might be avoided in any one community can be obtained by

comparing for each separate type of cancer the incidence in that community with the lowest reliable incidence that is recorded elsewhere. For this purpose, the calculation is best confined to figures for men and women under 65 years of age, because the data on older people are unreliable (*see also* Appendix C). The proportion of avoidable cancers in older people is best estimated indirectly (*see below*). For certain types of tumor we have also thought it wise to omit rates for those communities that are believed to have low rates largely because of genetic insusceptibility. Finally, we have omitted the common non-melanoma skin cancers entirely as, although they vary in incidence even more widely than most other types of cancer, reliable figures for their incidence are not generally available and they are, in any case, easily treated and seldom fatal.

Before incidence rates in different communities can be compared meaningfully, however, they must first be corrected for the fact that some communities have a higher proportion than others of young people (among whom cancer is everywhere extremely rare). This is allowed for by "age standardization," which we have done by calculating what the incidence in each community would have been expected to be if the proportions of young people in each had been the same as in the respondents to the 1970 U.S. census. Details are given in appendix A, and age-standardized rates for different communities can differ only if the incidence rates observed among people *of a given age* really differ between the different communities.

To estimate the proportion of all cancers that might have been avoided, we have taken, as an example, the population under 65 years of age in Connecticut during 1968–72 and have compared the incidence of each type of cancer (other than non-melanoma skin cancer) in that population with the incidence rates recorded in the populations listed in table 7. For example, the age-standardized rate for cancer of the esophagus among men under 65 years of age in Connecticut was 34.6 per million, while that in rural Norway was only 6.5 per million. Similar calculations were made for 37 other types (or groups of types) of cancer in men and for 40 types (or groups of types) in women. In selecting low rates, we confined ourselves to data from about 1968 to 1972 from registries selected by the IARC (1976) as being reasonably reliable.

The results are shown in table 7, and the total of these low incidence rates is contrasted with the corresponding totals for all types of cancer (except non-melanoma skin cancer) in Connecticut and in many other parts of the United States in table 8. The comparisons in table 8 suggest that in most parts of the United States in 1970 about 75 or 80% of the cases of cancer in both sexes might have been avoidable. The proportion could be more, as the lowest rates that have been used almost certainly include some avoidable cancers, especially since some of the countries that differ most markedly in various ways from the United States do not have a good cancer registry and so have not been used in table 7. (Moreover, the proportion in 1980 will probably be about one percentage point larger than that in 1970 due to the steady increase in tobacco-induced lung cancer in the United States.) However, the proportion that might by practicable means be avoidable may well be somewhat less than is suggested by tables 7 and 8, partly because in a developed area such as the United States some lumps may have been counted that, although histologically "cancer," were biologically benign (appendix C), but, more importantly, because even if means of modifica-

TABLE 7.—*Cancer rates[a] in selected low-incidence areas among people under 65 years of age[b,c]*

Type of cancer	Male rates in:		Registry with lowest reliable incidence for:		Female rates in:	
	Connecticut registry	Low-incidence registry	Males	Females	Connecticut registry	Low-incidence registry
Lip	11.8	4.1	United Kingdom, southern metropolitan region	United Kingdom, Birmingham	0.8	0.4
Tongue	19.8	4.1	New Mexico: Spanish	Israel: ♀ Jews	6.7	2.7
Salivary gland	7.3	2.3	Japan, Miyagi	Japan, Miyagi	6.7	1.2
Mouth	31.3	0.8	" "	" "	11.8	2.4
Oropharynx	13.9	1.1	" "	" "	6.0	0.8
Nasopharynx	5.6	2.4	East Germany	East Germany	1.1	1.1
Hypopharynx	10.7	1.4	" "	" "	2.9	0.2
Esophagus	34.6	6.5	Norway, rural	Norway, rural	8.3	1.8
Stomach	66.2	28.0	New Mexico: whites	United States, Iowa	26.7	16.6
Small intestine	6.4	3.0	Israel: Jews	Israel: ♀ Jews	5.0	2.5
Colon	137.2	13.7	Nigeria, Ibadan	Nigeria, Ibadan	140.7	11.6
Rectum	98.6	14.1	" "	" "	66.1	17.2
Liver	11.8	6.0	United Kingdom, southern metropolitan region	United Kingdom, Oxford	5.3	1.0
Gallbladder, plus ducts	9.0	3.3	Norway, rural	Norway, rural	11.2	6.7
Pancreas	45.1	21.0	Nigeria, Ibadan	Nigeria, Ibadan	30.9	14.9
Nose	3.2	2.2	United States, Iowa	United States, Iowa	2.4	1.5
Larynx	54.7	11.5	Japan, Miyagi	Japan, Miyagi	8.2	0.4
Bronchus	325.8	9.0	Nigeria, Ibadan	Nigeria, Ibadan	96.9	8.7
Bone	9.3	7.3	Puerto Rico	United States, Iowa	7.5	5.2
Connective tissue	20.0	12.5	United Kingdom, Birmingham	United Kingdom, southern metropolitan region	14.6	6.4
Melanoma	40.8	8.0	United Kingdom, Liverpool	United Kingdom, Liverpool	38.6	18.4
Breast	3.5	1.7	Finland	Israel: ♀ non-Jews	593.7	100.9
Cervix	—	—	—	Israel: ♀ Jews	90.4	42.5
Choriocarcinoma	—	—	—	United Kingdom, Oxford	1.2	0.2
Other uterine cancers	—	—	—	Japan, Miyagi	150.6	11.1
Ovary	—	—	—	" "	104.8	25.9
Other female genital organs	—	—	—	" "	16.0	2.3
Prostate	92.3	5.3	Japan, Miyagi	—	—	—
Testis	26.6	7.1	" "	—	—	—
Penis	2.0	0.2	Israel: Jews	—	—	—
Bladder	113.1	17.8	Japan, Miyagi	Japan, Miyagi	32.8	7.3
Kidney	59.6	9.0	Nigeria, Ibadan	Nigeria, Ibadan	23.2	2.5
Eye	4.3	2.0	Japan, Miyagi	Japan, Miyagi	4.3	0.5
Brain and CNS	54.9	12.2	" "	" "	35.2	8.9
Thyroid	12.4	3.6	United Kingdom, southern metropolitan region	United Kingdom, Oxford	34.0	8.8
Other endocrine cancers	2.5	1.4	Puerto Rico	Puerto Rico	2.2	0.6
Lymphosarcoma	39.8	13.1	" "	" "	25.5	6.4
Hodgkin's disease	37.4	6.2	Japan, Miyagi	Japan, Miyagi	28.1	3.5
Other reticuloses	11.3	1.8	Israel: Jews	Israel: ♀ Jews	7.6	1.9
Myeloma	15.1	1.8	Japan, Miyagi	Japan, Miyagi	9.6	3.3
Leukemia	57.9	40.8	New Mexico: Spanish	" "	41.1	36.3
Polycythemia	4.8	0.6	Japan, Miyagi	" "	1.6	0.3
All other cancers	89.9	33.7	New Zealand: whites	New Zealand: whites	74.6	23.5
Total, all cancers	1,590	321			1,775	408

[a] For all tumors except those of benign or unspecified malignancy and non-melanoma skin cancers (which, collectively, accounted for <2% of all cancer deaths in the United States in 1978).
[b] From IARC (1976).
[c] Annual rates/million people <65 yr old, standardized for age as described in appendix A.

TABLE 8.—*Comparison of total tumor incidence rates[a,b] observed in various American cancer registries, circa 1970*

Area in United States covered by tumor registry[d]	Male tumor incidence		Female tumor incidence	
	Observed	Minimal,[c] as % of observed	Observed	Minimal,[c] as % of observed
Alameda, Calif. (W)	1,589	20	2,103	19
San Francisco, Calif. (W)	1,668	19	2,137	19
Connecticut	1,590	20	1,775	23
Iowa	1,422	23	1,594	26
Detroit, Mich. (W)	1,498	21	1,737	23
New Mexico (W)	1,469	22	1,784	23
New York, upstate	1,372	23	1,481	28
El Paso, Tex. (W)	1,245	26	1,682	24
Utah	1,215	26	1,464	28

"Ten areas" from TNCS (a study covering a moderately representative tenth of the whole United States)

TNCS White	1,519	21	1,702	24
TNCS Non-white	1,906	17	1,721	24
TNCS White and non-white	**1,557**	**21**	**1,705**	**24**

[a] Annual rates/million people <65 yr old, standardized for age as described in appendix A.

[b] *See* table 7, footnote *a*, for excluded tumors.

[c] The total of the lowest reliable rates for each type of cancer listed in table 7 was 321 (♂) and 408 (♀), which is a crude indication of the minimal incidence that might be achieved.

[d] W = whites only.

tion of cancer risks can be identified, these may not be socially acceptable. This might obviously be a serious limitation if preventive measures had perforce to be limited to ways whereby different countries already differ, for affluent people will not be persuaded to adopt certain aspects of the life-style of the impoverished. But there may be many different simple or highly technical ways of preventing the same cancer (*see* subsequent sections), some of which have not been inadvertently adopted by any country with a good cancer registry, at least one of which ways may be both practicable and acceptable.

About half of the cancers diagnosed in the United States are found among people 65 or more years old, and we have made no explicit estimate in table 7 of what proportion of these might be avoidable. This is because data from cancer registries become very unreliable in old age, not so much in the United States nowadays as in those countries where the contrasts with the U.S. life-style and environment may be greatest. Consequently, any similar analysis of rates among older people might be severely biased. There is, however, little reason to suppose that the proportion of U.S. cancers that would be preventable differs greatly above and below the age of 65 years as long as lung cancer (which is relatively slightly more common among the old) and other cancers are considered separately (*see* section 5.1 and appendix E). Paradoxically, therefore, the most reliable available estimate of the proportion of cancer among older people that is

avoidable may simply be the proportion that is avoidable among middle-aged people.

The foregoing estimates refer to all malignant tumors, both fatal and non-fatal (excluding only non-melanoma skin cancer). Direct estimation by similar methods (but on the basis of national death certification rates instead of, as in tables 7 and 8, registered incidence rates) of the proportion of fatal cancers that are avoidable might be misleading. This is because many underdeveloped countries enumerate causes of death so inaccurately that comparison of their certified death rates from particular types of cancer with the corresponding rates in the United States might overestimate the proportion of U.S. cancer deaths that is avoidable. However, the two types of cancer (lung and large intestine) that currently kill the largest numbers of Americans have incidence rates that vary particularly widely between the United States and certain other countries and the U.S. deaths from these two types are therefore largely avoidable. The same is true of many other types of cancer that currently kill large numbers of Americans, and it is reasonable to suppose that the proportion of fatal cancers whose onset could have been avoided will be approximately the same as the avoidable proportion of all cancers discussed above, i.e., more than 75 or 80% in principle but perhaps less in practice for many years to come.

4. ATTRIBUTION OF RISK

4.1 Increases and Decreases in U.S. Cancer Rates

If there were currently an "epidemic" of cancer in the United States (by which we mean rapid increases in the probability of people *of a given age* developing most particular types of cancer), this might suggest that the search for avoidable causes for the cancers that we observe today should be directed chiefly toward various aspects of the modern environment that were much less widespread half a century or more ago. If, conversely, most of the cancers that are now common have been common for many decades, then, although this would not be evidence as to whether our new habits will eventually increase or decrease future cancer risks, it might suggest that the cancers that are currently common, and that will continue to be common unless we do something about them, have been largely determined by long-established aspects of the American life-style or environment.

Practical Difficulties in Gauging Cancer Trends

Cancer is certainly much more noticeable nowadays than it was a decade or two ago, but this is not in itself evidence that cancer rates are increasing as there are several factors that influence public awareness about cancer. First, especially when active treatment is being undertaken, the friends and relatives of cancer patients (or the general public, if the patient is a public figure) may discuss the disease openly, whereas previously such matters often used to be hushed up and the

TABLE 9.—*Death certification rates/1,000 Americans,*[a] *1935 and 1975*

Sex	Years	All causes except neoplasms		All neoplasms[b] except respiratory cancers		Respiratory tract cancers		All causes	
		Rate	%[c]	Rate	%[c]	Rate	%[c]	Rate	%[c]
Male	1933–37	15.12	91.0	1.42	8.5	0.09	0.5	16.63	100
	1973–77	8.91	81.0	1.41	12.8	0.69	6.2	11.01	100
Female	1933–37	11.92	87.6	1.65	12.1	0.03	0.2	13.60	100
	1973–77	4.96	78.8	1.17	18.6	0.16	2.5	6.29	100

[a] All ages, standardized for age to U.S. 1970 census (*see* appendix A). For most scientific purposes, separate examination of the trends above and below the age of 65 is preferable (*see* appendixes C and D), since many deaths from cancer half a century ago may have been miscertified as due to other causes, particularly among older people.

[b] Benign and malignant tumors are included in this table, as elsewhere throughout this text.

[c] Rate as percent of corresponding all-causes rate in last column.

diagnosis perhaps withheld even from the victim. Second, some cancers are now diagnosed that might previously have gone unnoticed in the medical treatment (and subsequent death certification) of dying people, especially of the elderly. Third, cancer has become *relatively* more common as a cause of death chiefly because of the prevention or cure of so many other diseases. This is nicely illustrated by the data for females in 1935 and 1975 (table 9). The non-respiratory cancer death rates decreased substantially, but the death rates from all other causes decreased even more substantially. Therefore, the *percentage* of female deaths attributable to non-respiratory cancer is actually greater now than it was 40 years ago, even though among women of a given age the *absolute* cancer risks are lower nowadays. If attention had been restricted to people under the age of 65 years (text-fig. 2), then the contrast between declining absolute rates and increasing percentages would have been even more marked. Fourth, there is a larger proportion of old people nowadays, and cancer risks are ten or a hundred times greater among old people than among young people. Finally, cancer has become a highly political issue, and consequently discoveries (perhaps using modern ultrasensitive analytical methods) of even quite small amounts of carcinogens in various everyday contexts attract vigorous media coverage, as do various other aspects of cancer research.

We shall therefore review in this section, and in our appendixes C, D and E, some of the objective evidence concerning the upward and downward trends in the U.S. death rates from, and incidence rates of, various cancers. Epidemic increases in lung cancer are clearly taking place, as would be expected as a result of the widespread adoption of cigarette smoking earlier this century, but apart from this we can see no good evidence of a cancer "epidemic" in the above sense.

Unfortunately, both cancer *registration* rates (a "cancer registry" tries to count all the new cancer onsets in a particular area, such as the State of Connecticut) and cancer *death certification* rates are subject to large

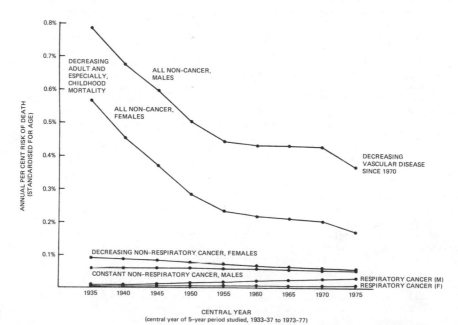

TEXT-FIGURE 2.—Annual age-standardized death rates, 1933–77, among Americans under 65 years of age.

errors; more unfortunately, these errors are not constant with time so that artifactual trends in the registered incidence or certified mortality rates for particular cancers may be superimposed on the true trends. The problem with any comparisons of cancer rates in different decades is that these artifactual trends may be of the same order of magnitude as the trends in real cancer onset rates that one wishes to study. The chief sources and likely magnitudes of such biases are discussed in appendix C.

Reduction of Bias: Trends in Mortality in Middle Age

The data suggesting moderate improvements in relative 5-year survival rates (e.g., from 60 to 68% for breast cancer) are also discussed in appendix C (*see* table C2 on page 1278), where it is suggested that part at least of these moderate apparent improvements is artifactual, due to progressively more complete enumeration of the non-fatal cases. Changes in treatment for many types of cancer have chiefly improved palliation rather than cure of the disease, and the true cure rates for many of the common types of cancer have probably changed very little since 1950. For these types of cancer the trends in death certification rates among people under 65 years of age, at which ages treatment of the curable and medical investigation of the causes of death of the incurable have for decades been reasonably careful, may paradoxically yield a much more reliable (and representative) indication of the real trends in cancer onset rates than can the superficially more attractive study of any of the currently available data on registered incidence rates. The need to restrict attention to death certification rates for people *under* the age of 65 years arises because many people who died of cancer in past years never had their disease diagnosed and might have been certified as dying of pneumonia, senility, or the wrong type of cancer. Progressive correction of such errors over the past several decades has resulted in large artifactual trends (some upward, some downward) in the death certification rates for certain types of cancer, especially during the first half of this century or, since 1950, especially among old people. (These and various additional biases also affect the trends in disease registration rates, where a registry tries to count both all fatal and non-fatal cases of cancer: *see* appendix C.) However, for most types of cancer the trends since the **1950's** among **middle**-aged American death certification rates seem likely to yield a reasonable indication of the true underlying trends in the corresponding real disease onset rates.

Increase in Middle-Aged Mortality From Respiratory Cancer

Either by examining the lower lines in text-figure 2 with a magnifying glass, or by referring to appendix tables D1 and D2 (pp. 1282–1283) from which text-figure 2 was derived, it can be seen that male respiratory cancer death rates appear to have been rising steadily for at least half a century and that female respiratory cancer death rates started to rise a quarter of a century ago and are now increasing alarmingly rapidly. The trends in respiratory cancer are discussed in more detail in appendix E, where we conclude that before 1950 almost the whole of the apparent increase in female lung cancer and some of the apparent increase in male lung cancer were artifactual, due to more accurate detection of lung cancer, but that some of the pre-1950 male increase and virtually all of the more recent increases in both sexes are real and are largely or wholly caused by the delayed effects of the adoption, decades ago, of the use of cigarettes (*see also* section 5.1). (The long delay between cause and full effect arises because even among people who have smoked regularly throughout most of their adult lives the degree of exposure of the lungs to cigarette smoke during their late teens or early twenties remains a surprisingly important determinant of lung cancer risks in middle or old age. *See* text-fig. E1 on page 1292.)

Lack of Generalized Increase in Middle-Aged Mortality From Non-respiratory Cancer

Text-figure 2 and tables D1 and D2 (pp. 1282–1283) also indicate that the aggregate of all non-respiratory cancers has taken a fairly constant toll among males for half a century (with about a 10% decrease among younger men in the past decade), but that the total non-respiratory cancer death rate among females has been decreasing rapidly for half a century, due not chiefly to improved treatment but rather to decreased onset rates among women of a given age. For age-specific details, *see* text-figs. C1 and C2 on page 1272. (All the overall comparisons we make are based on "age-standardized" rates, which can change only because of changes in the risk of cancer among people of a given age; increases or decreases in the proportions of old people will not affect them. This is not true of "crude" cancer rates nor of "percentages of all deaths attributable to cancer," and these should never be used to characterize trends: *see* appendix A.) However, non-respiratory cancer is an aggregate of many completely different types of cancer, some of which are increasing and some of which are decreasing.

Text-figures 3 and 4 describe, for males and for females, respectively, changes in mortality (or, more strictly, death certification rates) during the past quarter century for various types of cancer. More detailed data are presented in table D3 on page 1284, together with a separate discussion of the apparent changes in mortality from various particular types of cancer among people under 65 years of age. Corresponding details for people aged 65 years and over appear in table D4 on page 1285. All the changes are small in comparison with the large increases in the smoking-related cancers of the respiratory and upper digestive tracts, although the decreases in mortality from cancers of the stomach and uterus are also important.

In appendix D we also present the recent (1968–78) trends in death certification rates among Americans in

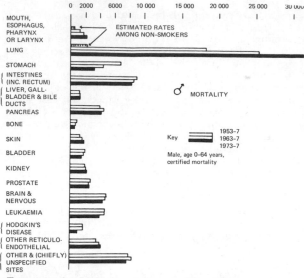

TEXT-FIGURE 3.—Certified mortality per 100 million males, ages 0–64 years (standardized for age to U.S. 1970 population as described in appendix A).

early middle life (35–44 years of age), as it is here that the first effects of any changes for better or worse in the causes of cancer might first be clearly evident. Reassuringly, no unexpected upward trends emerge (*see* table D6 on page 1287), while significant downward trends are seen in mortality from many types of cancer. For males, the sites where there are now significant decreases in mortality at ages 35–44 years include the pancreas, lungs (presumably chiefly due to decreasing tar yields per cigarette: *See* appendix E), and genitalia. For females, they include the intestines, genitalia, reproductive system, and breast (the latter decrease due perhaps to a protective effect of early childbirth on the mothers of the 1950's glut of babies). Overall, cancer mortality among young adults in the United States is decreasing quite rapidly, and much of the decrease cannot plausibly be attributed to improved therapy.

Trends in Incidence, as Assessed by Cancer Registry Data

Turning (with some trepidation, because of the greater likelihood of bias) from trends in certified mortality to trends in registered incidence, we are immediately confronted with the problem of exactly which incidence data to study—those from particular cancer "registries" that have operated for decades, trying to list all the cases, fatal or otherwise, of cancer in New York or Connecticut, those from comparison of the Second National Cancer Survey (SNCS) in 1947 or 1948 with the Third National Cancer Survey (TNCS) in 1969–71, or those from comparison of the TNCS with the Surveillance, Epidemiology, and End Results (SEER) program of the mid-1970's? (SNCS,

TNCS, and SEER all tried to monitor cancer incidence in about one-tenth of the entire U.S. population.) Unfortunately, many of the above comparisons suffer from such large artifactual irregularities and biases (*see* discussion in appendix C and text-figs. C3 to C5, pp. 1274–1276) that for most types of cancer they yield much less reliable information about long-term trends in real disease onset rates than the mortality data do.

The only one of these comparisons of cancer incidence rates that is at all compatible with the mortality data is that of the SNCS (in 1947 or 1948) with the TNCS (in 1969–71). This comparison has been described by Devesa and Silverman (1978, 1980). From their 1978 paper we have abstracted text-figures 5 and 6, describing the changes in registered incidence rates for each of the major types of cancer. The overall pattern of change indicated by these text-figures is, of course, roughly similar to that indicated by the mortality data, for this was why we selected this particular comparison of incidence rates for study. Consequently, we would not strongly disagree with anyone who argued that even the comparison of incidence rates in text-figures 5 and 6 is so uninformative that it would be preferable to rely chiefly on mortality data (although some of the striking differences between certain of the trends in incidence may be informative as, for example, the apparent decrease in cancer of the cervix but not of the endometrium).

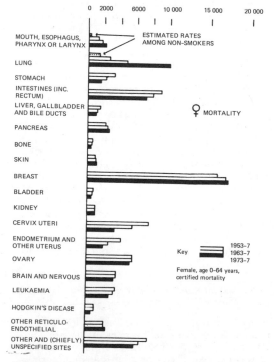

TEXT-FIGURE 4.—Certified mortality per 100 million females, ages 0–64 years (standardized for age to U.S. 1970 population as described in appendix A).

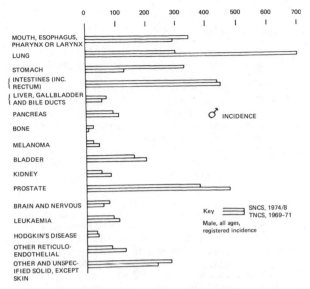

TEXT-FIGURE 5.—Registered incidence rates per million males, all ages (standardized for age to U.S. 1950 population and for race to 90% white).

However, even if the detail of the incidence trends is uncertain, the general picture is clear: *a*) the most important absolute increases have been in cancer of the lung, *b*) the most important absolute decreases have been in cancers of the stomach and uterine cervix, and *c*) less reliably, there seem to be no large changes in the aggregate of the incidence of all nonrespiratory cancer[9] (for which the age-standardized incidence registration rates decreased between 1947–48 and 1969–71 by 3% for males and by 19% for females.)

Comparison With Interpretations by Others

In summary, the trends since 1950 in mortality in middle age, somewhat reinforced by the trends in incidence between the Second and Third National Cancer Surveys, suggest that, apart from the effects of smoking (and perhaps asbestos: *See* section 5.6), there are no major epidemic increases in cancer. Unfortunately, our conclusion is not shared by all commentators. Epstein (1981b), whose book, *The Politics of Cancer*[10] (Epstein, 1978, 1979), was based on the

---

[9] We have excluded, since the surveys did not attempt to register it, non-melanoma skin cancer. Non-melanoma skin cancer is diagnosed more commonly than any other type of cancer, but it is nearly always so easily cured that it is one of the least common fatal cancers.

[10] For a wide-ranging comment on Epstein's (1978, 1979, 1981a, 1981b) perspective on the causes of cancer, which will make clear our reasons for not drawing on it in our present report, *see* Peto, 1980. The particular question of the role of occupational factors will be dealt with in section 5.6 and appendix F, where strong reasons for distrusting Epstein's (1981a,b) sources are given.

assumption that Americans live in an era of genuinely and rapidly increasing cancer rates over and above the increase due to tobacco, rejects it out of hand without acknowledging or explaining why the trend in U.S. mortality from non-respiratory cancer in middle age is actually downward, and without serious discussion of the potential biases in trends in death certification rates among older people (or, still more so, in trends in the registered incidence rates of tumors) that we have emphasized in appendixes C, D, and E. The Toxic Substances Strategy Committee (TSSC) in their 1980 report to the U.S. President also came to a conclusion directly opposite to ours, namely, that "even after adjustments for age . . . recent figures show that both incidence (new cases) and mortality (deaths) rates are increasing," and later that "when the effects of cigarette smoking are corrected for, the recent trends in incidence show an increase." Their conclusions about rising incidence rates were based on the data of Pollack and Horm (1980) and on the interpretation of these data by Schneiderman (1979) and rested heavily on a comparison of the incidence rates recorded in the TNCS during 1969–71 with those recorded in the ongoing SEER program that began in 1973. In appendix C we show that this particular comparison yields estimates of trends in real disease onset rates that are grossly discrepant with more reliable data.

An even more serious error in the TSSC (1980) report is the committee's peculiar method of "allowing" for the effects of cigarette smoking on the recent trends in

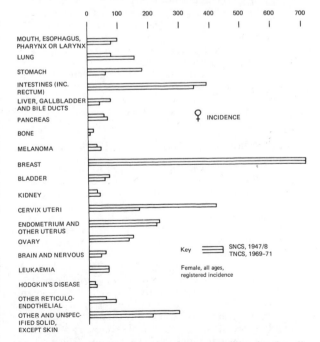

TEXT-FIGURE 6.—Registered incidence rates per million females, all ages (standardized for age to U.S. 1950 population and for race to 90% white).

lung cancer (and in certain other types of cancer) when it tries to estimate the residual effects of toxic substances other than cigarette smoke. The committee completely overlooked the fact that even if national exposure to cigarette smoke had remained constant throughout the 1960's and 1970's and all other relevant exposures had been constant throughout this century, large increases in lung cancer during this period would still have occurred due to the delayed effects of the large increases in cigarette consumption some decades before (*see* appendix E).

From this review of trends and from our more detailed review of trends in appendixes C, D, and E, we conclude that although a small part of the current morbidity from cancer may be due to new processes and products, it appears that changes in the American life-style, diet, or environment have also helped to reduce some old hazards, and (apart from lung cancer) most of the types of cancer that are common today in the United States must be due mainly to factors that have been present for a long time.

Implications

When seeking means to prevent cancer, we should certainly pay special attention to those types that are increasing in incidence, not only for fear that the increase may herald the onset of a new epidemic but also because the fact of the increase indicates that the cause (or causes) must have been introduced during this century and can presumably be eliminated. However, our review of trends obviously offers no guarantee that future risks may not be importantly affected by current exposure to some new factor(s) whose effects have yet to appear. To concentrate on a search for new agents to the exclusion of other causes is, however, to ignore the possibility of preventing that mass of present-day cancers which are due to avoidable factors that must have been prevalent in the Western world at least throughout this century or before.

4.2 Prediction From Laboratory Experiments

Over the past quarter of a century, various laboratory methods have been developed for predicting which particular chemicals would be likely to cause cancer if humans were acutely exposed to high doses or were chronically or intermittently exposed to low or moderate doses. An excellent review of the main methods and their relative merits has recently been compiled by the International Agency for Research on Cancer (IARC, 1980; *see also* Hollstein et al., 1979). The most favored methods now include not only "long-term" tests (in which the test chemical is usually fed at very high doses for a substantial part of the life-span of a few dozen rats or mice or some other small, short-lived animal to see if there is any marked excess of tumors of some particular type) but also various "short-term" tests, which are intended to be much quicker and cheaper than the long-term tests.

Different Types of Short-Term Test

The most attractive (IARC, 1980) short-term tests currently available fall into the following three main classes.

Effects on the genetic material (DNA) of cultured cells.—The test chemical may be applied, perhaps together with certain of the enzymes, etc., to which it would presumably be exposed in the human body (in case it is thereby "metabolically activated," i.e., converted from an inactive to an active form[11]), to suitably modified bacteria or mammalian cells growing freely in culture. The aim is to see whether the action of the test chemical or its metabolite(s), perhaps followed quickly by a round or two of cell replication, can cause the cellular DNA to suffer either a permanent change (i.e., one that is likely to be inherited by both daughters when changed cells divide and that can be detected by allowing selective proliferation of changed cells) or damage of a type which, although perhaps not directly detectable, causes particular cellular side effects[12] that can be detected. If bacteria are used (as in the "Ames test") then the whole test takes only a few days, but some important effects detectable only in mammalian cells may be missed, and vice versa. Even at the cost of somewhat increasing the number of "false-positive" findings, the use of both mammalian and bacterial short-term tests seems prudent for the more important chemicals.

Effects on DNA in the cells of living animals.—The test chemical may be administered in one very large dose to a few animals that are killed a few hours later, ground up exceedingly finely, and then examined (by alkaline elution) to see if the DNA extracted from any particular organ(s) shows breaks due to recent chemical attack. (Search in the urine of animals treated briefly with the test agent for excreted by-products of DNA repair has been proposed by various people but is not yet validated.) Alternatively, in the "mouse spot test," pregnant mice of appropriate genotype are treated with the test agent to see whether, 5 weeks later, their offspring will have a few spots on their fur due to chemical alteration in the fetal mice of the genetic information in a few single coat color cells (which proliferated during the intervening 5 weeks into a clone of descendants large enough to be seen as a spot of altered color). Finally, alterations in the sperm or other cells from animals may be sought. This latter technique, which is developing rapidly, may apply directly to putatively exposed human populations.

---

[11] No "metabolic activation" system seems perfect for use in short-term tests, but the most widely used system consists of microsomes extracted from fragmented cells from either rat or, preferably, human liver (IARC, 1980).

[12] Definitions of the side effects that may be sought, such as prophage induction, chromosomal "breakage," sister chromatid exchange, or "unscheduled" DNA synthesis, may be found in IARC (1980), but are not necessary for our present discussion.

Compared with tests on the DNA of cultured cells, tests on the DNA of cells in intact animals usually suffer from less uncertainty as to what form of metabolic activation is appropriate but more uncertainty as to the concentration of the test agent that reaches the target cells.

Effects on the behavior of cultured cells.—The test chemical may be applied (perhaps with some metabolic activation) to semi-normal cultured mammalian cells to see if it alters a few of them into cancerous-looking cells with a selective advantage, after a few weeks of growth in culture, over their unaltered neighbors.

Advantages of Short-Term Tests

The enormous advantage of the use of short-term tests is that they take only a few days or weeks and cost only a few hundred or a few thousand dollars (even if enough duplicate assays are done to achieve statistically reliable estimates of potency), whereas long-term tests take a few years and cost a few hundred thousand dollars (and the data may even then be subject to appreciable random or even systematic[13] statistical uncertainty unless a very striking carcinogenic effect occurs). Moreover, clear positive results in several short-term tests may yield the intangible but important benefit of conceptual clarification; for example, although we still do not know the cellular mechanism(s) whereby damage to DNA increases the likelihood of cancer, progress in understanding the mode of action of a carcinogen such as dimethylnitrosamine that damages DNA in many short-term tests is likely to be much more rapid than for carcinogens such as the halogenated hydrocarbons that are inactive in many short-term tests. Indeed, short-term tests have now developed to such a point that any serious scientific investigators who are responsible for initiating a careful long-term animal test on a particular chemical should themselves also routinely assume responsibility for ensuring that the results from the careful and competent execution of several short-term tests will be available to them before the final animal study report is prepared, for this increase of a few percent in the total amount spent will in most cases yield a very substantial increase in the scientific understanding of the biological effects of the test agent. No single short-term test can be relied on to pick up all effects of potential interest, which is why a combination of several such tests is advisable. (IARC, 1980, provides an excellent introduction to the selection of suitable short-term tests.)

Laboratory tests can be used either "exogenously" or "endogenously" to try to identify preventable causes of human cancer. First and most obvious, "exogenously," the additives, main components and contaminants of our drugs, drinks, diet, etc., may be separately screened in short- or long-term tests. Second, "endogenously," crude fractions of the feces (Bruce et al., 1979), blood, urine (Yamasaki and Ames, 1977), breast secretions, pancreatic juices, bile, etc. from several different individuals may be analyzed for moderate activity using some short-term method such as the Ames test which may be sensitive to very small amounts of active chemicals. If detectable activity is found in any sample, then that sample may be further fractionated in various ways, repeatedly using the short-term test activity as an assay to decide which fractions to throw away and which to subfractionate, until the active chemical(s) are located and characterized. Either before or after this, one may be able to experiment for a few days at a time with the few people whose fluids show the most pronounced activity, to find which aspects of their normal work, diet, drinks, drugs, diseases, medicaments, etc. chiefly determine the variation in total short-term test activity within individuals. Such findings may direct attention toward fruitfully testable specific epidemiological hypotheses which would not otherwise have occurred to the investigators.

Limitations of Short-Term Tests: Factors Affecting "Later Stages" of Carcinogenesis

From the above brief account of the nature and possible uses of laboratory cancer tests, it will be apparent that most of today's short-term tests rely heavily on the hypothesis that chemical agents which damage cellular DNA can cause cancer if they can gain access to the DNA in the "stem" cells of our bodies.[14] Most scientists find this claim plausible, but there is much less evidence for the converse claim that all of the really important determinants of human cancer are such agents. Quite apart from any possible inhibitors of carcinogenesis, there may be whole classes of chemicals that are human carcinogens but which are not likely to be detected by any of today's short-term tests.

---

[13] If, as is often the case, the test agent materially reduces the life expectancy of the heavily dosed group(s) of animals, then exact statistical correction for the effects of this on the yields of hepatomas or of any other moderately lethal type of tumor is impossible unless the cost-free precautions against bias recommended in the statistical annex to IARC (1980) are built into the conduct of the experiment. Omission of this may occasionally lead to unnecessary errors of interpretation of results which are of marginal statistical significance.

[14] The human body is composed of many cells that are incapable of any further division (e.g., many of the cells in our muscles, brains, and blood) plus many cells that appear capable only of a strictly limited number of further divisions, all the descendants of which will be inert or gone within the next few days or months, plus, most importantly of all, a few "stem" cells whose descendants will still be dividing a year or more hence and which are presumably the cells most at risk of cancerous alteration. Cairns (1975) has discussed the possible cellular basis of the differences between stem and other cells and has speculated that interference with the mechanisms which maintain these differences may be of critical importance in human carcinogenesis.

One fundamental reason for this is that alteration of a completely normal cell into the seed of a growing cancer may usually require at least two qualitatively different types of change, and the chief causes of one type may not be important causes of the other type, and vice versa (Peto, 1977, 1979). A cell that has undergone the "early" change(s) and is therefore now at risk of the "late" change(s) is, if it divides, likely to produce two daughter cells which are *both* at risk of the "late" change(s). So agents may in principle increase the likelihood of cancer in various completely different ways, perhaps by facilitating the early change(s), by conferring a selective advantage on partially altered cells relative to their normal unaltered neighbors, by facilitating the later change(s) (among partially altered cells descended from a stem cell that has undergone the early change(s)), or by interfering with any hypothetical host defense factors that may exist to restrain fully cancerous cells from proliferating.

Different cancer research workers tend to emphasize the relevance of different links in this chain, but none of the groups of processes are well understood. One class of chemicals called "initiators," which seem chiefly to affect the early stages, is reasonably well characterized, although the extent to which the "early" processes of the currently common human cancers are caused by such initiators is still unknown. Another class of chemicals called "promoters," which seem chiefly to affect either the selective proliferation of partially altered cells or the "late" processes (or, perhaps by separate mechanisms, both), is becoming reasonably well characterized, but again although promoters will undoubtedly be important tools for studying some particular mechanism(s) whereby cells *can* become cancerous, the common human cancer may not usually arise by such mechanisms (or, if they do, those mechanisms may have been triggered by accidents or agents unrelated to "promoters").

Perhaps the currently emerging understanding of "initiators" will turn out to be substantially correct, with the current short-term tests picking out all the important exogenous chemicals which currently cause human cells to undergo the "early" stages of carcinogenesis (and being useful tools in the search for the preventable determinants of the endogenous synthesis of such chemicals). However, "promotion" is still very poorly understood, as are almost all the other intracellular processes involved in transforming a partially altered cell into a fully cancerous cell. [One molecular biologist whose recent discoveries chiefly relate to "early," DNA-damaging carcinogens commented, "The key to carcinogenesis lies in understanding the later stages of the process; the early stages are just trivial molecular biology" (Cairns J: Personal communication). For review articles on the later stages of carcinogenesis, *see* Slaga et al., 1980.] Moreover, such "late" processes may turn out to be of much greater relevance to carcinogenesis in large-bodied animals like man that have to avoid cancer for 75 years than in the small, short-lived animals that laboratory workers must

necessarily study (Peto, 1979). If cells must independently undergo first "early" and then "late" processes before cancer can develop, then a 50% reduction in *either* class of processes would halve the eventual risk of cancer (Peto, 1977), and the only determinant of which class is more "important" is which is more easily halved.

Implications of, and Interrelationships Between, Results From Different Types of Tests

Some evidence bearing indirectly on the reliability of long-term tests comes from the correlation between the findings in mice and rats. Purchase (1980) found 248 compounds that had been tested in both species, and in each species about half these compounds were significantly carcinogenic and half were not. If the results in each species were of no predictive value whatever, one might expect 50% agreement and 50% disagreement by chance alone, whereas in fact Purchase found 85% agreement and only 15% qualitative disagreement.[15] However, the similarities between rats and mice are obviously greater than the similarities between rats and humans, so the percentage of correct answers if rat carcinogenicity were used to predict human carcinogenicity in a similar range of chemicals would presumably be less than 85%. (For comparison, remember that, given the real data on carcinogenicity among mice for each compound, deciding whether to call that compound "a rat carcinogen" merely on the flip of a coin should yield 50% "concordance" between the two species!) Considerably more direct evidence that both short-term and long-term tests are moderately reliable is provided by the observation that most chemicals that have been found to be carcinogenic in *both* rats *and* mice also exhibit marked DNA-damaging activity in one or more of the short-term bacterial mutagenicity tests, whereas most chemicals that have been tested and found not to cause any significant excess of cancers in *either* rats *or* mice are inactive in all such tests.[16]

---

[15] Some of these apparent discrepancies may have been due merely to chance fluctuations in the outcomes of certain particular experiments causing false-positive or false-negative results that would have been avoided had larger groups of animals been studied. Ideally, a mere tenfold discrepancy between the carcinogenic potency of a chemical in two different species should not be considered a qualitative discrepancy, although it might appear to be so if there were no statistically significant effect in the hardier species. Practically, however, the false-positives and false-negatives that inevitably arise by chance in realistic animal tests are an important inherent limitation of the method.

[16] The quantitative details of the correlations of results between short-term and long-term tests are subject to vigorous dispute (e.g., Ames and McCann, 1980; for a review and extensive bibliography, *see* IARC, 1980), which is why no percentages are cited. When there is eventual agreement as to how accurately short-term tests do predict which among a thousand particular chemicals are carcinogenic for rodents, it would be reasonable to hope for a similar degree of accuracy in predicting which of these thousand will be carcinogenic

Turning to more directly relevant correlations, of the 39 established human carcinogenic agents or circumstances which were listed in table 6 on page 1203 a mere *one third* are well-characterized individual chemicals which might have been picked up as clearly carcinogenic in *routine* feeding experiments in mice and rats, while the remaining two-thirds are not. Of those which are not, some are chemicals which although able to cause cancer in humans have not been found to be carcinogenic in any animal experiment thus far devised or have been found to be carcinogenic in animals only if given intrapleurally or subcutaneously, but not if given in their diet.[17] However, some of the factors listed in table 6 as affecting human cancer are not chemicals at all (e.g., various forms of radiation or immunosuppression, certain infective agents, and various physiological changes caused by pregnancy or hormonal alteration), although of course it is just as important to recognize these as to recognize carcinogenic chemicals. In others of the listed carcinogenic circumstances the responsible chemicals have not been identified with certainty (e.g., certain manufacturing processes and also two extremely important causes of human cancer, betel chewing and tobacco smoking). The study of cigarette smoke exemplifies the practical difficulties in using laboratory tests to predict human cancer risks. In developed countries tobacco may be the most important single cause of cancer, currently accounting for about one-third of all U.S. cancer deaths (section 5.1), but for many years cigarette smoke failed to produce malignant tumors in routine animal inhalation tests (a fact used in those years to deny the relevance of the human lung cancer data!). By persistent modification of the experimental circumstances malignant tumors were eventually produced by animal inhalation of cigarette smoke, and repeated application of certain components of cigarette smoke to the skins of laboratory mice can easily be shown to cause cancers. However, despite a quarter of a century of intensive study in a variety of animal and other laboratory systems, it remains unclear which of the many components of cigarette smoke "tar" are the most important causes of human cancer, and so the relative carcinogenicity for humans of tobacco "tars" of various different compositions cannot be predicted with confidence, nor can it be stated with confidence

that everything other than the "tar" is innocuous. (Likewise, cigarette smoke is an important cause of both vascular and respiratory disease, but for both the causative components of the smoke remain uncertain.)

On this evidence, animal feeding studies have great value in certain circumstances but may not offer an uncomplicated and straightforward means of discovering preventable causes for the majority of human cancers, and at the very least it certainly does not seem likely that they can offer a reliable means of estimating quantitative human hazards.

There is, however, an important sense in which examination of table 6 is not a fair way to assess the extent to which human carcinogens can be detected by routine rodent feeding tests on particular chemicals, for by definition table 6 excludes the greatest successes of animal feeding tests, i.e., the instances where these detect human carcinogens that epidemiology has not detected. (Nitrosamines exemplify this possibility.) But this may be counterbalanced by the fact that table 6 also excludes by definition any "false positives," i.e., agents which confer no material risk in the circumstances in which humans are exposed to them but which are significantly carcinogenic in laboratory animals, either due to random fluctuations[18] or due to important differences between mice and men. (Phenobarbital may be an example of such an agent: *See* Clemmesen and Hjalgrim-Jensen, 1977.)

Overlooking Important Determinants of Human Cancer

The trouble with all the foregoing attempted correlations, however, is that they depend rather critically on the range of chemicals that one chooses to study. Part of this trouble can be circumvented arithmetically [by expressing the results in terms of an "odds ratio" $(x/1-x)/(y/1-y)$, where x and y are the respective probabilities that agents active and agents inactive in a short-term test will be carcinogenic in a long-term test], but the more important troubles still remain. A nearly perfect screening system that picked up all currently known occupational carcinogens other than asbestos might be of less public health value than a lousy system that picked up asbestos but missed nearly everything else, simply because asbestos causes such a large percentage of occupational cancers. Likewise, a lousy research system that nevertheless identified one important preventable cause of breast cancer but which missed nearly everything else might be of more public health value for women than an ideal battery of long- and short-term tests for exogenous DNA-binding carcinogens. In other words, what we really need as the

---

to man, for the differences between bacteria and humans are not obviously greater than the differences between bacteria and small, short-lived laboratory animals (unless, to keep our large human bodies free of cancer for our long human life-span, we rely much more heavily than do rodents on some cellular mechanisms which have no analog in bacteria).

[17] Most insoluble dust particles that people inhale are ultimately transferred, via the respiratory tract mucus, down the digestive tract, so even for asbestos dust feeding studies might have been thought relevant but would probably have failed to detect the hazard. Studies of chronic inhalation of the various physical forms of dust to which humans are exposed would have discovered rat lung tumors in response to asbestos dust (Wagner et al., 1974).

---

[18] If statistical significance is assessed incautiously, the number of such "false positives" may be large, for in separate analysis of tumor rates in many organs in two sexes of two species many possibilities of a false-positive result will arise. For discussion of how moderate degrees of statistical significance in animal feeding tests should be interpreted, *see* the statistical annex to IARC (1980).

most relevant measure of the value of a laboratory test is a *weighted* correlation, in which the ability to predict the major ways whereby human cancer can be prevented counts for much more than the ability to predict minor causes and in which the identification of carcinogens to which humans are not and will not be seriously exposed is irrelevant.

Because this ideal measure of quality is unknowable, it is necessary to fall back on studying the correlations between the results of different tests, even though this may lead to a self-reinforcing over-valuation of the merits of the currently available test procedures. It is too soon to known which, if either, of the "exogenous" and the "endogenous" uses of today's testing technology will prove really fruitful in searching out previously unrecognized preventable causes of human cancer. Tobacco smoke is certainly active in many test systems, which is encouraging. But apart from tobacco, the avoidance of all human exposure to all the other exogenous and endogenous chemicals that are active in long-term animal studies or in today's short-term tests might have prevented surprisingly few of the cancers of today whose causes still elude us,[19] or perhaps avoidance of such exposure would have prevented most of them. Possibly, misleading conclusions are being drawn from over-emphasis on the spectrum of chemicals found active in mutagenicity tests and in chronic carcinogenicity studies in rodents. For example, the authors of official guidelines on how to do long-term tests usually emphasize the importance of concurrent controls and the need for strictly identical diet, handling, heat, light, stress, and infection in the treated and control animals. Why? Can minor details of the lifestyle of the animals really be important determinants of the animals' "spontaneous" tumor yields? And, if so, might not the same also be true for humans? In experimental animals, quite minor details of the total quantity of food and of the vitamins, fats, and carbohydrates (Jose, 1979; Roe and Tucker, 1974; Tucker,

1979; Conybeare, 1980; Roe, 1981) in the food can certainly be enormously important determinants of spontaneous tumor yields. But, because the mechanisms are not understood, short-term tests for the possible relevance to humans of these processes do not exist, and these phenomena are typically viewed as a potential nuisance to serious investigators who want to study the carcinogenicity of some trace environmental contaminant rather than as being themselves a potentially fruitful area of inquiry.

Difficulties in Quantitating Human Risks From Laboratory Data

Many promising lines of laboratory research into the development and use of various tests for carcinogenicity exist, but although there is every hope that current lines of laboratory research will draw attention to at least some of the preventable causes of human cancer, there is little reason to expect from them, at least in the near future, any *quantitative* predictions of human risk which are reliable to within a factor of ten or even, perhaps, a hundred. Quantitative extrapolations (e.g., of the dose in mg/kg/day which halves the lifelong probability of remaining tumorless) from animals to humans *may* already be giving us approximately correct assessments of human risk. Conversely, however, they may suggest risks that are wildly misleading in one or another direction. At present (*pace* Meselson and Russell, 1977) there seems to be quantitative human data on the risks from too few chemicals to know. The IARC (1980) review concluded that we are not even at the point yet where useful quantitative estimates of animal risk in long-term feeding studies can be derived from the findings in the various short-term tests, and, whether or not this is true, quantitation of human risk must therefore be a still more remote goal. Even if the potencies of different members of one particular family of chemicals are assessed for their activity in one short-term test and in one particular strain of animals, the correlation may be poor (Bartsch et al., 1980), so estimation of even the animal potency of a member of a previously untested class of chemicals may be still less reliable. Despite this unfortunate uncertainty, the quantitative data from laboratory tests (especially short-term tests) are, for many occupational, environmental, and dietary contaminants, the only information likely to be available in the next few years, and even tenfold or hundredfold uncertainties may be dwarfed by the millionfold variations between chemicals in their apparent potency and in the degree of human exposure to them.

Use of Laboratory Data for "Priority Setting" But Not for "Risk Assessment"

If our perspective on both short-term and animal tests is accepted, then quantitative human "risk assessment," as currently practiced, is so unreliable, suffering not only from random but also probably from large systematic errors of unknown direction and magnitude,

---

[19] Cairns (personal communication) has noted that exposure of the whole body of a smoker to a marked excess of Ames-test-positive mutagens (Yamasaki and Ames, 1977) results in only a moderate excess of urinary and pancreatic cancers and in no large excess of leukemias, lymphomas, or solid cancers at other sites distant from the respiratory tract. Cairns (1981) and German (1979) have also noted that although xeroderma pigmentosum patients are grossly defective in their ability to repair DNA damage due to almost all of the currently recognized Ames-positive mutagens, the very limited data available do not demonstrate an excess risk of cancer at any internal site. Finally, although the contents of the colon may be strikingly mutagenic in the Ames test (Bruce et al., 1979), this activity has not yet been evaluated as an important determinant of colon cancer, and since there can be similar mutagenic activity both in the human small intestine (where cancer is rare) and in the colons of many different species of animal, its significance remains open. It may turn out to be one of the most important observations yet made by any such methods, or alternatively if mutagenic feces have been common for millions of years then perhaps mammalian intestines have evolved effective defenses against them.

that it should definitely be given another name: "Priority setting" might perhaps be a more honest, although less saleable, name. So many thousands of chemicals are active to some extent or other in one laboratory test or another that it is difficult to know what, if any, practicable regulations to enact on the basis of laboratory tests. For some tests it has been recommended that the regulations which are promulgated should be based only on whether or not the chemical being tested is active, irrespective of the quantitative degree of activity of that chemical. But, if no explicit use is to be made of the degree of activity of each chemical, then instead of effective reduction of the total of all human cancer the chief result may be complete paralysis (either of the regulators or of the "regulatees").

A more proper use of each particular laboratory test might be to multiply the potency of each chemical studied in that test by whatever crude estimate is available of the degree of human exposure to that chemical, to yield some sort of index of human hazard according to that one laboratory test. When this has been done, it is likely that, for long-term tests and for each separate short-term test, one or a few chemicals will stand out head and shoulders above the rest with respect to these indices of human hazard. The best use of the various laboratory tests might be to identify, study, and if possible reduce these few apparently most extreme human hazards with respect to each particular test (together with any more moderate exposures that can be cheaply controlled) without necessarily requiring direct human evidence of harm. Although in many cases the benefits might be illusory, a few prudent restrictions against the apparent extremes with respect to each type of test might be nearly as effective as a broad action against all apparently active chemicals. This is true, however, only if before priorities are established a serious effort has been made to seek out as many sources of exposures as possible to agents active in that test (including endogenous formation of mutagens and other active agents in the gastrointestinal tract and exogenous absorption of such agents from involuntary or deliberate inhalation of smoke).[20] In the absence of direct evidence of the exact quantitative relevance to humans of the findings in long-term animal tests or in any of the short-term tests, blanket

restrictions on very large numbers of minor chemical pollutants may be unacceptably expensive, and the approach we have suggested might turn out to be a socially acceptable alternative way of setting a few priorities.

The conclusion that laboratory studies can be useful for priority setting but not for risk assessment is also prominently featured as one of the few major recommendations for change made by the National Academy of Science's recent committee of enquiry into the methods currently used by the Environmental Protection Agency to regulate pesticides (Committee on Prototype Explicit Analyses for Pesticides, 1980). Their thorough and thoughtful report addresses very nicely both the theoretical and the practical difficulties in regulating pesticides.

Returning to our present limited purpose of estimating the percentages of today's cancers that could be prevented by various particular means, we conclude that the great uncertainty inherent in quantitative estimation of human risks from currently available laboratory test results means that in what follows we must of necessity rely chiefly on quantitative epidemiological findings, merely reinforced in some of our final judgments about what is, and what is not, a real cause-and-effect relationship by laboratory findings.

4.3 Use of Epidemiological Observations

We concluded from previous sections that to estimate the percentages of current U.S. cancer deaths that might be avoidable in various ways, we must of necessity base our estimates chiefly on observations of the patterns of disease that are actually found in humans rather than on laboratory studies of particular chemicals, thus avoiding the many pitfalls, reviewed in section 4.2, inherent in extrapolation from laboratory studies to human experience. In this section we shall discuss some further advantages, disadvantages, and pitfalls of epidemiology. First, observations of the vagaries of human behavior may suggest ideas that might never occur to a laboratory investigator. Historically, they provided the starting point for a large part of all cancer research by pinpointing the risks associated with exposure to the combustion products of coal, sunlight, X-rays, asbestos, and many chemical agents. They drew attention to the hazards associated with chewing various mixtures of betel, tobacco, and lime and with smoking tobacco, and they suggested lines of research based on a hitherto unsuspected role for some type(s) of dietary fiber and on the relevance to breast cancer of the hormonal factors associated with pregnancy. Second, study of national trends in age-specific mortality from particular diseases may direct attention fruitfully toward diseases that are deserving of special further study (as happened in the 1940's with cancer of the lung), while study of the evolution of cancer rates among occupational or other groups in which an excess of cancer was present for reasons that were incompletely understood provides a monitoring system

---

[20] For example, in deciding how rigorously to regulate one particular source of environmental contamination by dioxins, it may be helpful to bear in mind the "background" extent to which such agents may be formed anyway wherever organic matter is burned (Bumb et al., 1980); in deciding how rigorously to regulate one particular source of dietary nitrosamines, it may be helpful to bear in mind the "background" extent to which nitrosamines are formed anyway in the human digestive tract (section 5.3); and in deciding how rigorously to regulate some other source of inhaled or ingested mutagens, it may be helpful to bear in mind the "background" extent to which the blood and urine of cigarette smokers are contaminated by such agents anyway (Yamasaki and Ames, 1977), for massive regulatory efforts against quantitatively unimportant targets may in their total effects be diversionary.

to check whether any hygienic measures that have been instituted have effectively reduced exposure to the actual causes of disease. Third, positive epidemiological observations (e.g., on radiation carcinogenesis) provide quantitative data relating directly to some of the doses to which humans are actually exposed. By so doing, they avoid or reduce the pitfalls in the extrapolation not only from one species to another but also from one dose level to another extremely different level and so provide estimates of the human risks associated with low exposure levels that are reliable enough for rational comparison of risks and benefits. Fourth, epidemiologists can sometimes study such large numbers of people that direct evidence of very small effects can be obtained. Humans feed themselves, house themselves, and arrange their own medical care at no cost to the epidemiologist. Observations can, therefore, be made on hundreds of thousands of individuals, whereas studies of comparable numbers of laboratory animals would be prohibitively expensive. No practicable experiment, for example, could have shown that doses of X-rays of the order of 1 rad to a fetus in its mother's abdomen could result in 1 cancer in every 2,000 individuals during childhood, as was shown in Great Britain by Stewart et al. (1958) and in the United States by MacMahon (1962).

Epidemiological observations, however, also have serious disadvantages that limit their value. First, they can seldom be made according to the strict requirements of experimental science, and consequently the available observations may be open to a variety of interpretations. A particular factor may be associated with some disease merely because of its association with some other factor that causes that disease, or the association may be an artifact due to some systematic bias in the information collection. Second, the observations that can be made on humans are limited to the conditions that have actually occurred. Except perhaps for the study of some putatively protective factor(s), the observations cannot be repeated at the command of the investigator with people exposed, for example, to another dose. Moreover, although large numbers of people may have been exposed to a moderate dose of some agent (e.g., an air or water pollutant), no comparable study groups may be available that have been consistently exposed to doses different enough for a measurably large difference in risk to arise (see below). Third, it may not be possible to detect the effects of a carcinogen on people until it has been in use for many years. Long induction periods are common for cancer, and hazards that are undetectably small after 10 years' exposure may be major after 30 years. By the time effects are clearly evident to the epidemiologist irreversible damage may have been done to large numbers of people, so that even after exposure is recognized and stopped cancers may continue to occur for many years.

These disadvantages limit the value of observations on humans, but they do not outweigh the major advantages that have been described. No one would choose to obtain evidence of the existence of a hazard by observing the appearance of a disease in humans if other practicable means were available, but until we know exactly how cancer is caused and how some factors are able to modify the effects of others, the need to observe imaginatively what actually happens to various different categories of people will remain.

Interpreting Epidemiology: Need for Comparison of Individuals, and Not Only of Large Groups

Trustworthy epidemiological evidence, it should be noted, always requires the demonstration that a relationship holds for individuals (or perhaps small groups) within a large population as well as between large population groups. Correlation between the incidence of cancer in whole towns or whole countries and, for example, the consumption of particular items of food can, at the most, provide hypotheses for investigation by other means. Attempts to separate the role of causative and confounding factors by the statistical techniques of multiple regression analysis have been made often, but evidence obtained in this way is, at best, of only marginal value.[21]

In practice, the danger of reaching a wrong conclusion from epidemiology is slight when observations are made on individuals rather than on whole populations and when the risk of disease is increased many times by exposure to the agent under suspicion. In these circumstances, risks have been detected that are quite small in absolute terms (affecting perhaps only one exposed person in 1,000) and some have been detected after only a handful of cases of a rare type of cancer have occurred in all.

Limitations of Epidemiology

The situation is, however, very different when the induced disease is as common as cancer of the lung or cancer of the breast is now. In these circumstances, human studies will be able to detect a specific risk only if the absolute risk of death is quite large. Even risks that will ultimately kill, for instance, 1% or more of the exposed population may be overlooked or attributed to chance unless a very large-scale investigation is undertaken. In these circumstances, too, when the cancer

---

[21] It is commonly, but mistakenly, supposed that multiple regression, logistic regression, or various forms of standardization can routinely be used to answer the question: "Is the correlation of exposure (E) with disease (D) due merely to a common correlation of both with some confounding factor (or factors) (C)?" The trouble is that unless the confounding factor is something (such as age or sex) that can be estimated with negligible measurement error, adjustment by any standard statistical techniques of the correlation of E with D for the *measured* values of C will reduce *but will not extinguish* the correlation between E and D even if, given the error-free (but unknown) values of C, no correlation between E and D would remain. (See appendix B14: Two properties of multiple regression analysis *in* Fletcher et al., 1976.) Moreover, it is obvious that multiple regression cannot correct for important variables that have not been recorded at all.

rates among exposed people are only a moderate multiple of those among the unexposed (e.g., when the relative risk lies between 1 and 2, as for kidney cancer among smokers or breast cancer among women who have been treated with reserpine; for an excellent discussion of the latter example, *see* Labarthe, 1979), problems of interpretation may become acute, and it may be extremely difficult to disentangle the various contributions of biased information, confounding of two or more factors, and cause and effect.

In short, unless epidemiologists have studied reasonably large, well-defined groups of people who have been heavily exposed to a particular substance for two or three decades without apparent effect, they can offer no guarantee that continued exposure to moderate levels will, in the long run, be without material risk. For this reason, prudent restrictions on occupational or public exposure to various substances often have to be based on indirect inference from laboratory studies of the agent being examined, without any direct evidence concerning its actual effect on humans. That is not to say that human evidence can ever be dispensed with. It is always relevant, but the weight that can be given to it varies greatly with the duration and intensity of the exposure experienced by individuals. Positive evidence (unless due to confounding) is always important. Negative human evidence may mean very little, unless it relates to prolonged and heavy exposure. If, however, it does, and is consistent in a variety of studies (correlation studies over time, cohort studies of exposed individuals, and case–control studies of affected patients), whereas the laboratory evidence is limited in its scope to, for instance, a particular type of tumor in a few species, negative human evidence may justify the conclusion that for practical purposes the agent need not be treated as a human carcinogen. In practice it is, of course, not usual for such perfect negative human evidence to be available, but even less conclusive negative human evidence may help determine priorities between different courses of action.

Advantages of Epidemiology

Our present purpose, however, is not to predict the future effect of new agents, but to make estimates of the proportions of today's cancers that are attributable to various avoidable causes, and for this purpose epidemiology, influenced by laboratory investigation, is far superior to the latter alone. Epidemiology has at present an undeservedly low reputation among people who have first artificially limited themselves to wondering which environmental pollutants to restrict and who then find that almost none of the few thousand chemicals they are worried about have been adequately studied by epidemiologists. This is, however, to condemn epidemiology for failing to achieve ends that it does not have. Epidemiology starts not with the 10,000 chemicals polluting a particular city but with the 10,000 annual cancer deaths in that city, and it tries to determine the major causes of these actual deaths. Epidemiology is, admittedly, more likely to overlook

many undetectably small effects of various chemicals than laboratory studies might do, but it is much less likely to overlook the large determinants of contemporary cancer rates and trends, especially if these are not simple environmental pollutants or dietary contaminants.

4.4 Shared Responsibility: Two Avoidable Causes of One Case of Cancer

Attribution of the risk of cancer to different causes is complicated by the fact that some agents interact with others to produce effects that are much greater than the sum of the separate effects of the same two agents. That synergism of this sort can be important has been known for more than 30 years. The experiments of Rous and Kidd (1941) and of Berenblum and Shubik (1947) indicated that the development of cancer in their experimental animals should be regarded as a process that could be accelerated by different agents acting at different periods, some of which had to act early on to "initiate" the process while others could act at a later stage to "promote" it (*see* section 4.2, but for modification of Berenblum and Shubik's 1949 evidence, *see* Stenbäck et al., 1981).

That the risk of human cancer might also be increased synergistically by the interaction of different agents has been suggested by a variety of studies of cigarette smokers who are also exposed to other agents. Stocks (personal communication; *see also* Doll and Hill, 1952) proposed it 30 years ago to account for the fact that the mortality from lung cancer in large British towns was about twice that in rural areas, despite the fact that the incidence in non-smokers was almost equally low in all areas. But whether cigarette smoking and atmospheric pollution do interact in this way still remains to be proved; the evidence is discussed in some detail in section 5.7. It is clear, however, that smoking may act synergistically in conjunction with ionizing radiations (Archer et al., 1976) or asbestos (Hammond et al., 1979; Saracci, 1977) to produce cancer of the lung and in conjunction with alcohol to produce cancers of the upper respiratory and digestive tracts (Tuyns et al., 1977; Herity et al., 1981). Finally, evidence is accumulating that some dietary factors, perhaps involving the consumption of β-carotene (Peto et al., 1981), may decrease the risk of cancer in several different parts of the body, including cancer of the lung among smokers (Bjelke, 1975; Hirayama, 1979). The evidence for this will be discussed in detail in section 5.3, but it is mentioned now to illustrate a principle (approximate multiplicativity of effects) that may have general applicability in the prevention of cancer.

If a variety of factors commonly interact to produce cancer, this may greatly facilitate prevention of the disease, but it complicates the attribution of risk. For if two different factors are each responsible for 75% of all cancers that occur at a particular site, in the sense that appropriate modification of either would result in a reduction in the incidence of the disease to a quarter of its previous level, we have a choice between two lines of action for preventing most cases, one of which may be simpler, quicker acting, or more acceptable than the other. In this situation, the additional effort required to modify both factors may have little absolute additional effect. Gratifying though this is to the specialist in preventive medicine, it means that if anyone tries to work out the extent to which human cancer is preventable by adding up the numbers of cases that could be prevented by various individual measures taken separately, it may look as if more than 100% of all cancers can be prevented! In the above example, for instance, we might appear to be claiming to prevent 150% of all cancers if anyone were to add the two proportions of 75% together.

This difficulty means that it is inappropriate to present a neat balance sheet adding up to 100% indicating the proportion of all cancers that are preventable by strategies X, Y, and Z. However, although cancer research may one day progress to the point where several separate ways are known of preventing each single case of cancer, it has not done so yet. Consequently, the amount of "double counting" in the estimates which we shall present of the proportions of present-day U.S. cancer deaths that can be prevented by various separate methods is small. We shall therefore ignore the anomaly in the rest of this paper and hope that, once it has been pointed out, no one will fall into the trap of adding together proportions that are not, in fact, mutually exclusive.

5. AVOIDABLE CAUSES

Information that would allow a direct quantitative attribution of risk to different aspects of the American environment or life-style is, for the most part, lacking. When it is available, we have used it. Otherwise, we have made estimates on the basis of extrapolations of uncertain reliability, clinical impressions, and contemporary hypotheses. In some instances, however, the evidence is so shaky that it is not justifiable to make any quantitative estimate at all. In this situation, scientific opinion about what is or is not justifiable will inevitably, and properly, vary, and it is through differences of opinion, subjected to testing by the validity of the predictions based on them, that advances are made. In the following sections we try at least to make clear those attributions that are reasonably firm and those that are semi-educated guesses.

We have based our estimates on the number of cancer *deaths* occurring each year in the United States, as it is deaths that we are seeking most urgently to prevent. Except for the very common non-melanoma cancers of the skin, which are usually easily cured, the percentages attributable to different factors would be altered only slightly by the inclusion of non-fatal cancers.

5.1 Tobacco

No single measure is known that would have as great an impact on the number of deaths attributable to cancer as a reduction in the use of tobacco or a change to the use of tobacco in a less dangerous way. The principal impact would be on the incidence of cancer of the lung, which by late middle age is more than ten times greater in regular cigarette smokers than in lifelong non-smokers, but a material effect would also be produced on the incidence of cancers of the mouth, pharynx, larynx, esophagus, bladder, probably the pancreas, and perhaps the kidney. This conclusion derives principally from studies in which a large number of people have been asked what they normally smoke and have then been followed for several years to determine the causes of any deaths that may occur among them. Table 10 presents data from the 16-year follow-up of one such study, and qualitatively similar findings have emerged from the other large U.S. study (Hammond et al., 1977), from our own study of mortality in relation to the smoking habits of British doctors (Doll and Peto, 1976), and in many other such studies in various countries (for reviews, *see* Surgeon General 1979, 1980, 1981).

The conclusion that cigarette smoke is a direct cause of cancer derives from many different types of epidemiological evidence (Surgeon General, 1979), combined with the fact that the smoke can cause cancer in experimental animals. For a good early review of the evidence and a spirited rebuttal of various rather foolish (but common) counterarguments, *see* Oettlé, 1963. Since the ratio of the lung cancer mortality rate in regular cigarette smokers to that in lifelong non-smokers is so extreme, it follows (*see* section 4.3) that cigarette smoking must be a cause of all, or nearly all, of the excess of lung cancers observed among smokers. This conclusion incidentally accounts nicely for the striking increases in lung cancer mortality that have been observed in recent decades among the males and then among the females in many countries (*see* table 5 on page 1202), including the United States (appendix E) and for the decreases in lung cancer among younger American men that have just begun to emerge during the 1970's (text-fig. E3 on page 1295) following the decreases in cigarette tar yields during the 1950's and 1960's.

By contrast, the difference in incidence between smokers and nonsmokers is less marked for cancers of the bladder, pancreas, and kidney than for cancers of the respiratory or upper digestive tracts, but the accumulating evidence suggests that an average consumption of cigarettes approximately doubles the incidence of cancer of the bladder and probably also of the pancreas, while being associated with a more moderate increase in kidney cancer. That smoking should affect bladder cancer and perhaps kidney cancer is not surprising, since tobacco smoke contains a wide variety of mutagenic and other chemicals, some of which are absorbed from the lungs into the bloodstream, circulate through distant organs, and are found at particularly increased concentration in the urine of smokers (Yamasaki and Ames, 1977).

TABLE 10.—*Comparison of numbers of deaths observed[a] among a sample of male U.S. cigarette smokers[b] with the numbers that would have been expected if their rate of death had been the same as that of age-matched[c] non-smokers*

Certified cause of death	Deaths by mid-1970 of men who in the 1950's were current smokers of cigarettes only			
	No. of deaths observed	No. expected from corresponding non-smoker experience[c]	Difference between observed and expected	Ratio of observed to expected
Cancer				
Lung	2,609	231	2,378	11.3
Mouth, pharynx, larynx, or esophagus	452	65	387	7.0
Bladder	326	151	175	2.2
Pancreas	459	256	203	1.8
Kidney	175	124	51	1.4
All other cancers[d]	3,660	2,796	864	1.3
Total, all cancers	**7,681**	**3,623**	**4,058**	**2.1**
Other causes				
Respiratory disease[e]	2,107	488	1,619	4.3
Cardiovascular disease[f]	21,413	13,572	7,841	1.6
Other certified causes[g]	3,721	2,564	1,157	1.5
Cause not available[h]	1,221	610	611	2.0
Total, all causes	**36,143**	**20,857**	**15,286**	**1.7**

[a] In the 1950's, a quarter of a million U.S. veterans described (once only) what they smoked; the certified cause of death was sought for any of these veterans who died in the 1950's and 1960's [Rogot and Murray (1980)].

[b] Of those who described themselves in the 1950's as current cigarette smokers, a) some had smoked cigarettes for only a *part* of their previous adult lives; b) even among smokers the mean consumption of cigarettes before 1945 was probably lower than in the 1950's, and c) some of the 1950's smokers subsequently gave up smoking. Consequently, the excess of lung cancer and of any other diseases that can be caused by smoking would be even more extreme than in this table among men who had smoked one pack of 20 cigarettes/day fairly regularly (without giving up) ever since *early* adult life (*see* appendix E, text-fig. E1, page 1292).

[c] Standardized for single years of attained age. For details, *see* Rogot and Murray (1980).

[d] Including leukemias, lymphomas, benign tumors, and tumors of unspecified site or malignancy. Some smoking-related cases of lung cancer may have the site of origin unspecified or mis-specified on the death certificate. This accounts for some of the excess mortality observed among smokers from cancers in this aggregate "all other" category.

[e] Excluding tuberculosis (81 deaths observed vs. 36 expected). Most of the excess mortality from respiratory disease was actually *caused* by smoking [Fletcher et al. (1976)].

[f] Some, and perhaps most, of the excess mortality from cardiovascular disease was caused by smoking [Doll and Peto (1976)].

[g] Some, but by no means all, of the excess mortality from other certified causes was actually caused by smoking.

[h] Either because the certified cause was incompletely specified, or, more commonly, because the death certificate was not located by Rogot and Murray (1980).

Different Types of Tobacco and Ways of Smoking

The ill effects of smoking are much greater when tobacco is smoked in the form of cigarettes than when it is smoked in other ways. This is probably not because of any special effects of burning paper or of cigarette tobacco additives but may be because, compared with the smoke from pipes or cigars, cigarette smoke is less alkaline.[22] The difference between cigarettes and other forms of tobacco is most marked in regard to lung, bladder, and pancreatic cancers and less marked (if it exists at all) in relation to cancers of the mouth, pharynx, larynx, and esophagus. The effects of

---

[22] The alkalinity of pipe or cigar smoke may so facilitate absorption into the bloodstream of the nicotine which some smokers need that sufficient quantities of nicotine can be absorbed while pipe or cigar smoke is merely held in the mouth, without any need for inhalation deep into the lungs. Moreover, alkaline smoke from pipes or cigars is more irritating than cigarette smoke and so again is less readily taken into the lungs.

different types of cigarettes may likewise differ from each other, and it appears that today's low-tar cigarettes may in the long run prove materially less harmful (Hammond et al., 1977; Wynder et al., 1976) than the cigarettes of a quarter of a century ago. For lung cancer (though not necessarily for all other tobacco-associated diseases) the risk reduction may be 50% or better (*see* appendix E), to judge by the rapid decreases in male lung cancer now being seen in Britain, but reliable data, especially on the effects of *long*-term use of various low-tar cigarettes, are still not available. [*See*, however, Gori and Bock (1980), Surgeon General (1981), and Lee and Garfinkel (1981) for a review of the epidemiology to date.]

Quantitative Attribution of Risk

Our present purpose is to estimate the percentages of U.S. cancer deaths in 1978 that were caused by tobacco, i.e., the percentage of deaths that would have been avoided if the individual had not smoked. We shall do this by estimating separately the numbers of deaths from each separate type of cancer (lung, larynx, bladder, etc.) that were caused by smoking. Our chief sources of data are *a*) the male and female age-specific death rates from each cancer among all Americans in 1978; *b*) the corresponding death rates (Garfinkel, 1980) observed during 1959–72 among half a million Americans who in 1959 said they had never smoked regularly and whose subsequent mortality was monitored by the American Cancer Society (ACS); and *c*) some approximate information about national smoking habits. Three main approaches are possible, and we shall first discuss them in relation to lung cancer.

The first, and probably the best, method is to assume that the male and female age-specific death rates from lung cancer observed among the ACS non-smokers in 1959–72 would have applied to the whole country in 1978 if no one had ever smoked, to work out how many U.S. lung cancer deaths would thereby have been predicted ($\approx$12,000), and, since there were actually some 95,000 lung cancer deaths in the United States in 1978, to ascribe the excess ($\approx$80,000–85,000 lung cancer deaths) to tobacco. One great virtue of this method is that it automatically allows for any effects on cigarette-induced mortality of the switch to low-tar cigarettes and of any other changes in national smoking habits. This method does suffer from some sources of uncertainty, but none seriously affect the final estimate. Perhaps the lung cancer death rate among non-smokers has increased between the 1960's and the 1970's (Enstrom, 1979a; Schneiderman, 1979b), although we consider that the evidence does not support this conclusion (appendix E). Alternatively, perhaps the ACS follow-up was slightly biased. Certainly, the diagnostic accuracy in the ACS study was different from the 1978 national average, if for no other reason than because all deaths certified as being due to "cancer" during the first half of the study period were specially investigated, and a few that had been miscertified as lung cancer were reclassified as other cancers, and vice versa. Finally, perhaps the ACS non-smokers (who, in addition to having chosen not to smoke, were probably of somewhat higher socioeconomic status than the nation as a whole) differed in some important personal characteristics from the nation as a whole, although no plausible personal characteristics which are important determinants of lung cancer among non-smokers are yet known.[23] Because of all these possibilities, the prediction of "about 12,000" is subject to at the very most twofold uncertainty (and in our view rather less), but even so the true number of lung cancer deaths in the United States in 1978 if no American had ever smoked

would have been somewhere between 5,000 and 20,000 (although the range 10,000–15,000 seems considerably more probable). However, on subtraction from the 95,000 national total these uncertainties become less important, and we are confident that in 1978 between 75,000 and 90,000 of the deaths certified as lung cancer were caused by tobacco. (The annual number of lung cancer deaths ascribable to tobacco is, of course, not stationary at $\approx$83,000 but is increasing by $\approx$4,000 per year as the lung cancer epidemic evolves.)

This estimate of 12,000 refers, of course, to the total number of lung cancer deaths per year that would have occurred in the absence of tobacco, and not to the number that currently occur among non-smokers. Indeed, since most Americans in middle or old age are either smokers or ex-smokers and only about 20% are lifelong non-smokers, the above estimate of 12,000 suggests that the annual number of lung cancer deaths per year among lifelong non-smokers must currently be only a few thousand [i.e., about 2 or 3% of the annual total of about 100,000 U.S. lung cancer deaths, and certainly nowhere near the figure of 20% (!) suggested by Epstein and Swartz, 1981].

This same (first) method is applied to respiratory, upper digestive, bladder, and pancreatic cancers in table 11. The results[24] suggest that there would have been only about 40,000 deaths attributable to these four types of cancer in 1978 if no American had ever smoked, instead of the 155,000 or so that actually occurred.

The difference ($\approx$115,000) represents, in our view, a fairly reliable estimate of the number of U.S. deaths from these four types of cancer that were caused by smoking in 1978. To it we have added a few thousand deaths certified as due to other specific types of cancer (*see* notes to table 11), yielding a grand total of about 120,000 or 125,000, i.e., about 30% of all U.S. cancer deaths. A very slightly higher figure might be more plausible, as we have probably underestimated the numbers of smoking-related cancers miscertified as occurring at other specified or unspecified sites. However, the range of reasonable uncertainty about our estimate is quite narrow and would not include a figure as low as 90,000 (since our estimate would still exceed 100,000 even if the associations of smoking with pancreatic or bladder cancer were eventually discredited, and we have not assumed any specific effect on kidney cancer) nor a figure as high as 150,000 (since our estimate would still be less than 140,000 even if fully 10% of the quarter of a million remaining cancers were attributed to smoking, a proportion approximately double that suggested by the differences between smokers and non-smokers in the ACS data).

The whole of this first method, of course, depends on the accuracy with which the death rates recorded

---

[23] A personal characteristic which is well established as a determinant of cancers of the mouth, pharynx, larynx, and esophagus is alcohol consumption (*see* section 5.2), and we must try to allow for the likelihood that the ACS non-smokers drank less than the U.S. national average when we come to estimate the numbers of U.S. deaths from these particular types of cancer that were actually caused by tobacco. However, there is no evidence that alcohol consumption has any direct effect on lung cancer.

---

[24] Augmented by 7%, since 7% of all people certified as dying of cancer do not get the site of origin specified on the death certificate (*see* table 11).

TABLE 11.—*Cancer deaths caused by tobacco: United States, 1978*

Certified cause of death[a]	No. of deaths		
	Observed	Estimated, had Americans not smoked	Approximate excess attributed to tobacco
Cancer, males			
Lung	71,006	6,439[b]	64,567
Mouth, pharynx, larynx, or esophagus	14,282	1,792×2[c]	10,698
Bladder	6,771	2,960[b]	3,811
Pancreas	11,010	6,585[b]	4,425
Other specified sites	100,799	?	5,000?[d]
Unspecified sites	14,469	8,188[e]	6,281
Total, males	218,337		94,782 (43%)[f]
Cancer, females			
Lung	24,080	5,454[b]	18,626
Mouth, pharynx, larynx, or esophagus	5,100	1,458×2[c]	2,184
Bladder	3,078	2,170[b]	908
Pancreas	9,767	7,291[b]	2,476
Other specified sites	127,642	?	1,000?[d]
Unspecified sites	13,951	11,879[e]	2,072
Total, females	183,618		27,266 (15%)[f]
Total, males and females	401,955		122,048 (30%)[f]

[a] Site of origin of cancer.
[b] Number estimated by applying the nonsmoker mortality rates reported by Garfinkel (1980) to the U.S. population of 1978.
[c] Double the number estimated by the procedure described in footnote *b*. This number was doubled to allow for the possibility that the subjects in the ACS prospective study were less exposed to alcohol (*see* section 5.2), or to some other cause(s) of cancer of the upper respiratory or digestive tracts than were average people in the United States. [Some evidence that this was indeed the case is that even the cigarette smokers in the ACS study had mortality rates for these types of cancer that were somewhat below the national U.S. rates: Hammond (1966).] However, it makes little difference to our grand totals whether the small number of cancers of the mouth and throat "expected" from the ASC nonsmoker experience are left unaltered, are doubled, or are trebled.
[d] Other specified sites include some, such as kidney, which may truly be affected by tobacco, and some, such as stomach or liver, that include a proportion of misdiagnosed cases of cigarette-induced cancer of the lung, pancreas, and other organs. Some fraction of the cancers certified as being of other specified sites is thus due to smoking, which in part explains the excess mortality among smokers in the aggregate of all such cancers that is found in the American prospective studies (*see* table 10). We have suggested, without firm evidence, that of these other cancers, perhaps 5,000 ♂ and 1,000 ♀ cases may have been due to tobacco. These suggested figures, totaling 6,000, may slightly underestimate the actual figures, but readers may substitute any estimate that they consider more plausible, e.g., some other estimate between 1,000 and 20,000, leading to an estimate of 29–34% of 1978 cancer deaths ascribable to tobacco.
[e] Estimated to match the proportions (43% ♂, 15% ♀) of specified sites attributed to tobacco.
[f] The percentage ascribable to tobacco is gradually increasing as lung cancer death rates are increasing among old Americans.

among non-smokers in the ACS study during the 1960's are representative of the death rates among non-smokers in the general population during the late 1970's,[25] and for bladder cancer at least there is in-

dependent confirmation that the correspondence is reasonably good. Analysis of the data from the large case–control study of Hoover et al. (1980) would predict some 5,500 bladder cancer deaths in 1978 if nobody had smoked, which is within 10% of our prediction (table 11), based on the ACS non-smoker rates, of 5,130. Likewise, both in the study of a quarter of a million U.S. veterans (Kahn, 1966) and in our own study of British doctors (Doll and Peto, 1976; Doll et al., 1980) the numbers of deaths from the aggregate of cancers of the lung, the upper respiratory and digestive tracts, the bladder, and the pancreas observed among the non-smokers were within 10% of what would have been predicted from Garfinkel's (1980) report of the ACS experience, which again supports the general applicability of the ACS rates to other non-smoking populations. Finally, we note that the ACS female non-smoker rates for cancer of the lung are rather similar to the rates that prevailed among U.S. women as a whole in 1950, before the epidemic increases in cigarette-induced lung cancer began to affect women.[26] Thus these low rates could indeed prevail among the population as a whole were it not for tobacco.

A second, much less satisfactory, method is to assume that the male and female age-specific excess lung cancer death rates observed among the ACS smokers in 1959–72 would have applied to all U.S. smokers in 1978. Not only are there known to be large differences in the lung cancer rates between smokers in 1978 and smokers a decade or two earlier, but also, just as importantly, uncertainty in the absolute risks among smokers would cause very wide uncertainty in the number of deaths attributed to smoking if this second method were used. In contrast, some uncertainty in the absolute risks among non-smokers does not cause wide uncertainty in the number of deaths attributed to smoking by our first method.

A third method would be to assume for each category of cancer that the percentage excess rate observed among smokers in the ACS study will be similar to the percentage excess among smokers in the country as a whole. The possibility of error (especially since, for bladder and pancreatic cancers as for lung cancer, the percentage excess is probably increasing from one decade to the next) is obvious, but for cancers for which only a twofold risk is associated with smoking, the near-twofold uncertainty about the ab-

[25] Strictly, of course, we would like to estimate the lung cancer death rates that non-smokers would have had in the late 1970's if they had not even been exposed "passively" to other people's cigarette smoke (*see* below).
[26] The annual lung cancer death rates per 100,000 women aged 45–54, 55–64, and 65–74 years were 5, 15, and 29, respectively, among ACS non-smokers (Garfinkel, 1980) compared with 7, 14, and 25 among all U.S. females in 1948–52. (*See* appendix E, tables E1 and E2. By 1950, the standards of diagnosis and cure for lung cancer were reasonably comparable with those of today, but no large effects of tobacco on female death rates were yet evident.)

solute rates for non-smokers inherent in the first method would obviously not have the negligible effect that it has on the numbers of lung cancer deaths attributed to smoking, and so for cancers other than cancer of the lung this method might be preferred in principle. However, for the four main categories of smoking-related cancer in table 11, it yields estimates so similar to those from the first method that we have not presented it in detail, although we note that it yields slightly higher estimates than those in table 11 for the numbers of "other and unspecified" cancers attributable to tobacco.

Potentially Biased Estimates

Finally, we have not made use of any data from the U.S. National Mortality Surveys (Enstrom, 1979a; Enstrom and Godley, 1980), as we suspect that data on smoking obtained from the relatives of dead patients may misclassify substantial numbers of ex-smokers as lifelong non-smokers, thereby overestimating the likelihood of cancer among non-smokers (for further discussion, *see* appendix E).

Nor have we considered the extent to which "passive smoking" (i.e., the inhalation of air polluted by other people's smoking) might affect the incidence of cancer either among smokers or among non-smokers. If the ACS non-smoker death rates during 1959–72 were materially higher than they would have been in the absence of the effects of passive smoking, then we may have slightly underestimated the total number of deaths due to tobacco, though the relative error must be small. However, whether or not there were appreciable effects of passive smoking on non-smokers during the 1960's, any effects on non-smokers (and, perhaps, on smokers) of passive smoking may eventually grow to be surprisingly large as the carcinogenic effects of tobacco smoke depend so strongly on the duration of exposure to it (Doll and Peto, 1978) that lifelong exposure (including childhood) may have four times the effect of exposure which is limited to adult life. In view of this, the twofold excess risks already reported merely among the non-smoking wives of cigarette smokers are disturbing (Hirayama, 1981; Trichopoulos et al., 1981, but for further data *see* Garfinkel, 1981).

Our estimate of 30% relates to the entire U.S. population and is somewhat higher than the estimate (22%) made by Hammond and Seidman (1980) of the percentage of the cases of cancer in the ACS study population itself that were attributable to smoking perhaps because a disproportionate number of the ACS cigarette smokers stopped smoking and partly because there are substantially more lung cancer deaths nowadays than 10 years ago. Conversely, our estimate is slightly lower than the figure of 38% that can be estimated from the tables presented by Enstrom (1979b).

*Future Changes in the Percentage of Cancer
Deaths Due to Tobacco*

While, as now, U.S. lung cancer death rates continue to rise, our estimate of the percentage of cancer deaths caused by smoking will likewise increase and will therefore probably be at least 33% by the mid-1980's, assuming no large trends in net mortality from non-respiratory cancer. How far it will ultimately rise and whether it will fall rapidly thereafter depend largely on whether current decreases both in sales-weighted tar yields and in cigarette consumption can be maintained or improved on, and for obvious reasons these cannot be predicted reliably. Indeed, even given knowledge of what (if any) deliberate increases in the cost of cigarettes, deliberate decreases in the advertising of cigarettes (or perhaps of cigarettes with 15 mg or more of tar), or deliberate increases in public awareness of the quantitative dangers of cigarettes will be brought about by the U.S. Congress, reliable prediction of their effects on the consumption of various types of cigarette would not be possible. In Canada, increases in cigarette price have coincided with decreases in cigarette consumption (Forbes, 1978), but strict proof of causality is, of course, lacking. In the United States, the Surgeon General's first (1964) report and the widespread discussion of the dangers of smoking that have followed it coincided with the start of a substantial decrease in the percentage of men who describe themselves as cigarette smokers (51% in 1965 vs. 37% in 1979; Surgeon General, 1980) and of a smaller decrease among women (33% in 1965, 28% in 1979). Even though cigarette sales have not decreased nearly as strikingly as this (appendix E), these changes suggest that worthwhile decreases in cigarette consumption can take place even without government really trying, but whether they were indeed due chiefly to public awareness of the hazards of smoking and whether they could be improved on by fostering more accurate public awareness of those hazards are simply not known. Therefore, although we can estimate reasonably accurately the present percentage (30%) of cancers due to smoking and can forecast an increase by two or three percentage points by the mid-1980's whether or not effective anti-smoking action is taken, longer term prediction is impossible.

5.2 Alcohol

It is convenient to consider alcohol next, not because it is the second most important cause but because it "interacts" with smoking, each agent enhancing the other's effects. That alcohol is involved in the production of cancer has been suspected for 60 years, since it was shown that cancers of the mouth, pharynx, larynx, and esophagus were commoner than average in men who were employed in trades that encouraged the consumption of large amounts of alcohol; and it has been confirmed subsequently in many detailed studies of men and women affected by these diseases in Europe and North America. Now, too, there is good evidence to suggest that alcohol consumption sufficient to cause cirrhosis of the liver will also increase the incidence of liver cancer. Precise figures for the proportions of these various cancers attributable to the consumption of alcohol have, however, not been easy to obtain, because an accurate account of the amount of alcohol an individual drinks is difficult to obtain and interpretation of any results has been further complicated by the fact that total abstainers are commonly distinguished by other behavioral characteristics (including avoidance of tobacco, which directly affects most of the types of cancer with which alcohol consumption is associated).

Much effort has been expended in trying to find out whether the effect of alcoholic drinks is due to the alcohol itself or to other chemicals that can be found in spirits, wines, and beers and whether it depends on the concentration of alcohol in the drink. Some evidence suggests that the effect is greatest when alcohol is consumed in spirits, and some suggests that the apple-based drinks consumed in Northwest France are particularly harmful; however, the totality of the evidence suggests that the principal effect is due to the alcohol itself and is largely independent of the form in which it is drunk, a conclusion reinforced by the observation of oral cancer among habitual users of strongly alcoholic mouthwashes (Maclure and MacMahon, 1980).

Both in Western Europe and in North America the carcinogenic effect of even quite substantial consumption of alcohol is small in non-smokers, increasing the incidence of cancers of the mouth and pharynx some two to three times (Rothman and Keller, 1972). In smokers, on the other hand, as is shown in text-figure 7, consumption of the same amount would have a larger absolute effect, as it seems to multiply the carcinogenic effect of tobacco smoke on the mouth,

pharynx, larynx, and esophagus, although it has no such effect on the lung (Wynder and Bross, 1961; Tuyns et al., 1977; Herity et al., 1981). Cancers of those sites related to alcohol consumption account for 7% of all cancer deaths in men and 3% in women. If we attribute about two-thirds of the former and about one-third of the latter to alcohol and add a small proportion of the liver cancer deaths (which constitute less than 1% of all cancer deaths), we arrive at an attributable proportion of about 3% of all deaths in both sexes. The range of uncertainty in this estimate is quite narrow and it is most implausible that the true percentage lies outside the range of 2–4%. It must, however, be emphasized that this figure cannot be added to the proportion attributable to tobacco because the two proportions largely overlap. In other words, most of the 3% of cancer deaths now caused by alcohol could have been avoided by the absence of smoking, even if alcohol consumption remained unchanged.

Pure alcohol is not by itself carcinogenic by any of the animal experiments thus far devised (which emphasizes the unwisdom of basing one's beliefs about human cancer too closely on laboratory studies), and although alcohol may have some direct effects on the genetic material of cultured cells (Harsanyi et al., 1977; Obe and Ristow, 1979), it seems possible that it exerts its carcinogenic effect in humans chiefly by facilitating contact between extrinsic carcinogenic chemicals and the contents of the stem cells that are responsible for the integrity of the lining of the upper digestive tract and larynx.

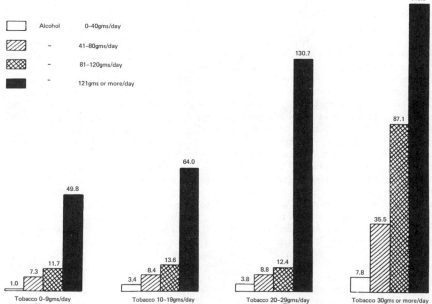

TEXT-FIGURE 7.—Relative risk of developing cancer of the esophagus in relation to smoking and drinking habits (redrawn from Tuyns et al., 1977).
Note that these data do not distinguish between non-smokers and light smokers, thus they do not indicate directly what the effects of alcohol would be among lifelong non-smokers.

TABLE 12.—*Some currently promising hypothetical or actual ways or means whereby diet may affect the incidence of cancer*

Possible ways or means	Paragraph No. in text	Example[a]
1. Ingestion of powerful, direct-acting carcinogens or their precursors	1(a)	Carcinogens in natural foodstuffs (plant products)
	1(b)	Carcinogens produced on cooking
	1(c)	Carcinogens produced in stored food by microorganisms (bacterial and fungal)
2. Affecting the formation of carcinogens in the body	2(a)	Providing substrates for the formation of carcinogens in the body (e.g., nitrites, nitrates, secondary amines)
	2(b)	Altering intake or excretion of cholesterol and bile acids (and hence the production of carcinogenic metabolites in the bowel)
	2(c)	Altering the bacterial flora of the bowel (and hence the capacity to form carcinogenic metabolites)
3. Affecting transport, activation or deactivation of carcinogens	3(a)	Altering concentration in, or duration of contact with, feces (fiber)
	3(b)	Altering transport of carcinogens to stem cells (alcohol?)
	3(c)	Induction or inhibition of enzymes (which affect carcinogen metabolism or catabolism)
	3(d)	Deactivation, or prevention of formation, of short-lived intracellular species (e.g., by use of selenium, vitamin E, or otherwise trapping free radicals; by use of β-carotene or otherwise quenching singlet oxygen; by use of other antioxidants)
4. Affecting "promotion" of cells (that are already initiated[b])	4(a)	Vitamin A deficiency (clinical or subclinical)
	4(b)	Retinol Binding Protein (hormonal and other factors determine blood RBP, though vitamin A intake may not affect it much)
	4(c)	Otherwise affecting stem cell differentiation (carotenoids? determinants of lipid "profile"?)
5. Overnutrition	5(a)	Age at menarche
	5(b)	Adipose-tissue-derived estrogens
	5(c)	Other effects

[a] There may be considerable overlap between many of the entries in this table.
[b] Or, more generally, affecting the probability that a partially transformed stem cell will become fully transformed and will proliferate successfully into cancer.

5.3 Diet

Diet is a chronic source of both frustration and excitement to epidemiologists. For many years there has been strong but indirect evidence that most of the cancers that are currently common could be made less so by suitable modification of national dietary practices. This is even more plausible now than it was 10 years ago, but there is still no precise and reliable evidence as to exactly what dietary changes would be of major importance. The chief need is, therefore, for continued and more intensive research. In humans both observational evidence and, perhaps, randomly controlled evaluation of the more promising hypotheses may be needed. In animals, the many mechanisms whereby dietary factors may influence cancer risks need to be understood, and the various dietary factors that do influence cancer risks need to be identified, even if their mechanisms remain obscure, as clear animal findings may suggest new questions for human studies to address.

Because reliable information is scarce, we shall describe the few components of diet that seem definitely carcinogenic, and we shall also review what seem to us to be some of the more promising current lines of research into both causative and protective agents. (Protective agents may be of more practical importance

than causative agents, for it may be easier to prescribe than to proscribe dietary factors.) Finally, we shall try to estimate very crudely the size of the benefit that might be expected if some of the results of current research live up to the expectations that many investigators have for them, but on present knowledge the range of permissible estimates must be very large.

The ways in which diet can influence the development of cancer are legion (Doll, 1979), particularly if "diet" is interpreted to include everything that is put into the mouth and swallowed. We shall use "diet," however, in a more limited sense and interpret it to mean only those items that occur in natural food or are produced during the normal processes of storage, cooking, and digestion. Chemicals that are mixed with food and drink to preserve them or alter their color or taste are considered separately in section 5.4 and those that are added unintentionally as a result of the agricultural use of pesticides, industrial pollution, etc., will be considered in section 5.7.

Even in this more limited sense there are still many completely different ways in which diet might act, several of which have only recently come to be considered as potentially significant in relation to the development of cancer in humans. Some of these are listed in table 12.

Of course, what ultimately matters from a public

health point of view is not so much the *mechanisms* whereby dietary factors may affect cancer, but rather the *nature* of the dietary factors that are important determinants of cancer. (Likewise, it is more important to know that cigarettes cause lung cancer than to know the mechanisms of this effect, although the great advantage of a mechanistic approach, of course, is that if mechanisms can be understood then this may lead to the study of agents which enhance or inhibit those mechanisms.) When the science of nutrition and cancer matures, it will be possible to redraft table 12 as a list of important protective factors and causes instead of as the present list of possibly important mechanisms. Indeed, there are already some dietary factors, such as fiber or β-carotene, where the hypothesis that they are protective is being studied directly in humans (either by uncontrolled epidemiology or by randomized intervention) while more than one mechanism whereby they might act is entertained in the laboratory. Conversely, there are some other dietary factors, such as overnutrition (which can greatly affect cancer risks in laboratory animals and may also affect human cancer risks), for which no mechanisms have been convincingly established. Such factors do not fit naturally into the classification scheme of mechanisms in table 12, despite their possible importance to humans. This underlines certain drawbacks of a mechanistic approach to the avoidable causes of disease. However, because the science of diet and cancer is immature, we shall adopt, as a framework of paragraph headings within which to review current and future research directions, the list of mechanisms in table 12, presenting the relevant epidemiology within this framework even though epidemiology always points to agents rather than to mechanisms.

1. Ingestion of Powerful, Direct-Acting Carcinogens or Their Precursors

1 (a) Carcinogens in natural foodstuffs.—The simplest and most obvious, although perhaps not the most important, dietary mechanism is the ingestion of small amounts of substances that are themselves powerful direct-acting carcinogens[27] in laboratory animals or which are converted into such carcinogens by metabolism in the body. Such substances include cycasin in the cycad nut, pyrrolizidine alkaloids in *Senecio* and some other plant genera, safrole in sassafras, and extracts of coltsfoot and bracken fern. Only the last has

been related to cancer in humans, Japanese who eat bracken fern daily appearing to have three times as great a risk of developing cancer of the esophagus as have Japanese who avoid it (Hirayama, 1979). The consumption of bracken fern is common only in Japan, and the naturally occurring carcinogens thus far recognized cannot be regarded as a significant cause of cancer in the United States. This may, however, be because a thorough search of foodstuffs for naturally occurring carcinogens is not yet complete, while the search for "co-carcinogens" and "promoters" is even less advanced. Dozens of natural foodstuffs can be tested one by one for their influence on animal cancer rates (e.g., uncooked soya flour predisposes rats to pancreatic cancer: McGuinness et al., 1980), but such experiments are laborious and may be insensitive, and any observed effects may be due to the gross disturbance of the diet (*see* below) rather than to trace carcinogens. The use of short-term tests may help by drawing attention to candidate substances, e.g., quercetin, a mutagenic (Tamura et al., 1980) natural substance which may cause cancer in animals (Pamukcu et al., 1980), the precursors of which are present in tea, red wine, bracken fern, and particularly, onions (Sugimura and Nagao, 1979). Although current short-term tests may overlook some carcinogens, particularly those that do not bind directly to the genetic material of the cells at risk (*see* section 4.2), laboratory discoveries of active agents may provide hypotheses specific enough for fruitful epidemiological inquiry. However, it is not yet clear whether any powerfully active substances are present in significant quantities in the natural components of the modern American diet.

1 (b) Carcinogens produced on cooking.—Another possible source of such substances is the production of carcinogens by cooking. Humans are the only animals that cook their food, and it has been known for many years that benzo[a]pyrene and other polycyclic hydrocarbons can be produced by pyrolysis when meat or fish is broiled or smoked or when any food is fried in fat that is used repeatedly. More recently, Sugimura et al. (1977) have demonstrated that pyrolysis of food (e.g., in charcoal-broiling steaks) also produces powerful mutagens that cannot be accounted for by the production of benzo[a]pyrene alone. Good cooks, however, do not usually *pyrolyze* much of the food they are cooking, although they may *caramelize* it. The chemical changes occurring during this more normal cooking procedure (which involves temperatures of only 100–200° C) have been insufficiently studied, but there is already evidence (Stich et al., in press; Spingarn et al., 1980) that various completely different chemicals are thereby produced that can damage or fragment cellular genetic material, both in cultured cells and in the intestinal tract (at least of mice).

Many epidemiologists have sought to relate the consumption of various cooked foods to the development of gastric cancer, but none have succeeded in doing so convincingly. Only Dungal and Sigurjonsson (1967) have obtained any human evidence that is even suggestive, and that is extremely weak. Few people eat

---

[27] Committees of experts have argued for so many hours over the precise definition of a "carcinogen" that we shall merely adopt Humpty Dumpty's strategy. What *we* mean by it is anything which, given under suitable experimental conditions in *small* quantities, causes a *substantial* risk of cancer, e.g., powerful initiators, powerful promoters, or anything that is efficiently converted into them in vivo. Our terminology is loose but may suffice until much more is known about mechanisms of carcinogenesis. With our definition, nitrosamines are "carcinogens," but nitrites are not.

more broiled food than Americans, and gastric cancer is rapidly diminishing in incidence in the United States. The method of cooking could be important, perhaps to some type of cancer other than gastric cancer, but at present this is unproven.

1 (c) Carcinogens produced in stored foods by microorganisms.—A less obvious source, and indeed one that was overlooked altogether until the early 1960's, is the production of carcinogens in stored food by the action of microorganisms. There is now good reason to believe that aflatoxin, a product of the fungus *Aspergillus flavus* that commonly contaminates peanuts and other staple carbohydrate foods stored in hot and humid climates, is a major factor in the production of liver cancer in certain tropical countries. Experimentally, it is among the most powerful liver carcinogens known for some animal species, and it is likely also to be carcinogenic for humans because human liver cells contain the enzymes needed to produce the particular metabolic products that appear to be responsible for its activity. It is, moreover, now clear that the incidence of primary liver cancer, which is the commonest type of cancer in inhabitants of large parts of Africa, is in those parts approximately proportional to the amount of dietary aflatoxin (*see*, for example,. Linsell and Peers, 1977). In all countries the disease occurs more commonly in people whose livers are chronically infected with the hepatitis B virus than among their uninfected compatriots, and it seems probable that, where aflatoxin is present in substantial quantities in the diet, both aflatoxin and hepatitis B virus contribute to the risk of liver cancer, each multiplying the other's effects.

The vagaries of daily diet and the short half-life of aflatoxin within the body make it unlikely that we shall ever be able to establish the relationship in individuals in the same way as a relationship was established between lung cancer and cigarette smoking, and it is difficult to see what further evidence could be obtained short of trying to reduce aflatoxin contamination of various foods in tropical areas to see if the disease would begin to disappear within one or two decades.

In the United States, primary cancer of the liver is a rare disease accounting for less than 1% of cancer deaths in people under 65 years of age. At older ages the diagnosis is often inaccurate (fatal cancers of other sites which have spread to the liver being miscertified as primary liver cancers), and the statistics are, therefore, unreliable. The amount of aflatoxin in the U.S. diet is minute, and it is only one among several possible causes of those few cases that do occur. It may, therefore, be questionable whether the return to be anticipated from rigorous attempts to eliminate all aflatoxin from the diet would justify the effort, although it would certainly be prudent to make reductions (particularly in retail nuts and nut products and in dairy products that have been affected via contaminated cattle feed: MAFF, 1980) if these could be achieved without disproportionate expense. In an Amer-

ican context, however, the chief importance of the discovery of the dangers of aflatoxin may be that it raises the possibility that other mycotoxins in food may be carcinogenic. None have yet been clearly demonstrated to be so in any country, but fusarial infection of stored food may contribute to the high incidence of esophageal cancer in parts of China, which reemphasizes the need to seek such agents elsewhere. (Miller and Miller, 1979, in a wide-ranging review of naturally occurring chemical carcinogens that may be present in food, particularly emphasize the possible dangers of fungal contamination by aspergillus, penicillium, or fusarium.)

2. Affecting the Formation of Carcinogens in the Body

2 (a) Providing substrates for the formation of carcinogens in the body.—Another possible mechanism that has aroused particular interest is the formation of N-nitroso compounds in the body. These are among the most powerful chemical carcinogens in the laboratory, and the production of even small amounts in the human body could be important. They are present in small amounts in the resting gastric juice and may be formed in the digestive tract or possibly in the infected bladder by a reaction between *nitrites* and various *nitrosable compounds* (secondary amines or N-substituted amides). The reaction is assisted by formaldehyde or by thiocyanate ions (perhaps from tobacco smoke), but it requires either a mildly acid medium or bacterial assistance and is inhibited by the presence of antioxidants (e.g., vitamin C) in the stomach.

This way of synthesizing carcinogens in vivo is of particular interest because neither nitrites nor nitrosable compounds can easily be avoided. Nitrosable compounds occur naturally in many foods, particularly in fish and meat; they may be ingested as pesticide residues or drugs, and they may be formed in the colon from amino acids. Nitrite may be derived directly from food, to which it has been added as a preservative or color and flavor enhancer, or in which it has been formed by bacterial action on nitrates, or it may be formed in the body by bacterial action on nitrates in the salivary ducts, the hypoacid stomach, and the infected bladder, and possibly on nitrates or nitrogen in the gut. The most important source of nitrite appears to be its production in vivo from nitrate, which is ingested in vegetables and, to a lesser extent, in drinking water and in foods to which nitrate has been added as a preservative. The relative importance of these different sources of nitrite are reviewed by Fraser et al., 1980. The possible role of meat and vegetables as dietary precursors of N-nitroso compounds was illustrated by the observation (Fine et al., 1977) that after a meal that included both bacon and spinach, blood levels of N-nitroso compounds rose sharply. There are, therefore, many ways in which carcinogenic N-nitroso compounds might be formed and many factors by which their formation might be modified. The questions that now must be answered are whether the amounts produced correlate with the incidence of any type of cancer in whole populations and, much more importantly, whether within populations they correlate with the risk to the individual.

The fragmentary evidence from epidemiology, which is reviewed by Fraser et al. (1980), chiefly relates to cancer of the esophagus and cancer of the stomach, but in neither case have clear positive findings emerged. Drinks and foodstuffs associated with cancer of the esophagus have been examined minutely for nitrosamines, with no clear positive results. Some relationship between gastric cancer and the nitrate content of the diet has been suggested, particularly in Latin America, but the relationship is not consistent. The much-cited example of the high mortality from gastric cancer in a British town where the water supply contained an unusually high concentration of nitrate (Hill et al., 1973) can be explained on the grounds that coal miners, whose gastric cancer rates are anyway likely to be high, constitute a high proportion of the resident population (Davies, 1980). It is notable that vegetables, which are usually the main source of dietary nitrates, appear if anything to protect against the development of gastric cancer (and of various other types of cancer, e.g., MacLennan et al., 1977, and many other studies). There is thus little evidence that dietary nitrates, nitrites, or nitrosable compounds contribute to the production of gastric cancer or any other type of cancer, but this may merely be because there is inadequate evidence on the whole subject.

2 (b) Altering intake or excretion of cholesterol and bile acids.—One way in which certain fats might contribute to the production of carcinogens in the body is by increasing the amount of bile acids and cholesterol metabolites in the feces. The evidence to support this suggestion has been reviewed by Reddy et al. (1980a) and is now substantial. In brief, larger amounts of these substances, and particularly of deoxycholic and lithocholic acids, are found in the stools of populations on a Western-type diet in whom colorectal cancer is common than in populations on characteristic African or Asian diets in whom it is rare. Larger amounts are also found in the stools of patients with cancer or adenomatous polyps in the colon than in the stools of patients with other diseases or of healthy controls. Moreover, the amounts in the stools can be increased experimentally in humans by high-fat, high-meat diets. In laboratory experiments on rats, high-fat diets (with various different fats) increase the fecal excretion of the same group of bile acids and increase the incidence of colon cancer induced by a variety of carcinogens, including 1,2-dimethylhydrazine and methylnitrosourea, and the same effects on cancer incidence can be obtained by feeding cholestyramine, a nonabsorbable resin that increases the excretion of bile salts.[28] Also, dietary cholesterol (Cruse et al., 1978) or

bile acids fed or administered intrarectally for a prolonged period to animals have a synergistic effect with the effects of small doses of carcinogens on the incidence of tumors of the large intestine.

Despite these observations and experiments, however, the relevance to human cancer of fecal cholesterol remains uncertain, for although dietary cholesterol ultimately reaches both the blood and the feces, there is no evidence that the levels of any form of cholesterol in the blood are correlated with the risk of developing cancer. On the contrary, there is some evidence to suggest that people with a low blood level of cholesterol suffer a higher mortality from cancer in a variety of sites. This finding has only recently been reported, and it is uncertain whether the association is an artifact, due to the effect of an undiagnosed cancer on the body's metabolism, as Rose and Shipley (1980) suggest, or whether it is real, as is suggested by the larger body of data collected by Feinleib et al. (1980). Even if the association is real, it may be coincidental and not causal. One way in which a coincidental association might be produced is through an association between the blood levels of cholesterol and of vitamin A (Young, 1976; Kark et al., 1980), the possible protective effects of which are discussed later on in this section. Conversely, one way in which a real association in either direction might in theory be produced is through the fact that some biologically active fat-soluble substances share with cholesterol a common vehicle of transport in the blood and of uptake by many types of peripheral tissue cell (i.e., the complex and specific system of fatty "low density lipoprotein" particles that contain much of the extra-cellular blood cholesterol, vitamin E, β-carotene, and other types of provitamin A.)

2 (c) Altering the bacterial flora of the bowel.—If cholesterol and bile acids are relevant, it may be because they are acted on by the bacteria in the colon to produce carcinogens that either act locally or diffuse elsewhere in the body. Likewise, many other chemical reactions can be effected by these bacteria, and a variety of diseases may perhaps be affected by any factor that determines which bacteria flourish in the large intestine and in what relative proportions. Unfortunately, the extrinsic determinants of the intestinal flora are poorly understood.

---

[28] Analogously perhaps, in a randomized trial of the prolonged human use of clofibrate, a drug which removes cholesterol from the bloodstream via the bile duct, a significant excess of cancer deaths among the clofibrate-treated patients was reported (Committee of Principal Investigators, 1978). However, a) although the excess of the aggregate of all types of cancer was statistically significantly higher in the treated than in the control group, none of the differences in any of the separate types of cancer were clearly significant and b) clofibrate itself is carcinogenic in animals, but it appears to act by a mechanism which has no direct connection with its effects on cholesterol (Reddy et al., 1980b). Thus even if clofibrate really is a human carcinogen, this may tell us nothing about the relevance to human cancer of cholesterol.

3. Affecting Transport, Activation, or Deactivation of Carcinogens

3 (a) Altering concentration in, or duration of contact with, feces.—One factor that may affect the bacterial flora which has recently received considerable attention is dietary fiber. Burkitt (1969) observed that several intestinal diseases that are common in developed countries are rare in rural Africa and India, where unprocessed food is consumed and the stools tend to be soft, bulky, and frequent, and suggested that dietary fiber might be important. This hypothesis was not at first supported, so far as colorectal cancer was concerned, by international statistics correlating food supplies with cancer deaths, but the figures that were available for fiber related only to crude fiber.[29] Since then, however, much work has been done to characterize the various components of dietary "fiber" as defined in Trowell's (1972) sense, which is remnants of the cell wall not hydrolyzed by human alimentary enzymes. Fiber in Trowell's sense is about five times as plentiful as crude fiber in, for example, whole wheat and contains lignins that pass through the bowel unchanged, cellulose that is partially degraded (50%) by bacteria in the large bowel, and hexose, pentose, and uronic acid polymers that are largely degraded (85%). All these, it now appears, have different effects. The pentose polymers in particular are mainly responsible for the production of soft, bulky stools, not so much because of their water-binding capacity, as was at first thought, but by increasing the population of certain intestinal bacteria. (A surprisingly large part of the bulk of a typical stool consists of intestinal bacteria.)

Food tables have now been prepared specifying separate amounts of the various different components of fiber in certain foods, and Bingham et al. (1979) have used these tables to correlate the mortality from colon and rectum cancer in the different regions of Great Britain with each fiber component. The results show a close inverse correlation between the pentose fiber content of the diet and mortality from cancer of the colon (but not of the rectum) which persists when each of the other dietary constituents studied is taken into account, and no correlation with any of the other types of fiber when the pentose fiber content is allowed for. (No good correlation is observed with dietary fiber as a whole, nor with vitamin C, fat, or beef.) As with all geographic correlations, however, the interpretation of these findings will remain uncertain until the relevance of the separate components of dietary fiber has been assessed directly in case–control or other studies on individuals rather than on whole populations.

Pentose polymers are particularly abundant in unrefined cereal fiber and to a lesser extent in various other vegetables (although not in potatoes), and case–control studies suggest that patients with cancer of the large bowel tend to have had a below average consumption of certain such vegetables (Modan et al., 1975; Bjelke, 1978). It could also be that the pentose polymer content of cereals will account for the correlation observed in Scandinavia between bulky stools and low colorectal cancer incidence. (In rural Finland, where large amounts of unrefined rye bread are eaten, the stools are bulky and the incidence of colorectal cancer is low, whereas the opposite is true in Copenhagen where the chief difference from the Finnish diet seems to be a much smaller consumption of unrefined cereals: IARC Intestinal Microecology Group, 1977.)

If some particular component of dietary fiber does reduce the risk of colorectal cancer, it might do so by decreasing the length of time stools remain in the bowel, by decreasing the concentration of carcinogens in the stools (through increasing their bulk), or perhaps by altering the total numbers or proportions of different bacterial species in the bowel, some of which may produce or destroy carcinogenic metabolites.

3 (b) Altering transport of carcinogens to stem cells.—Alcohol (*see* section 5.2) has been suspected of acting by affecting the transport of carcinogens, and presumably other dietary factors might likewise do so.

3 (c) Induction or inhibition of enzymes.—In laboratory animals, carcinogens that depend on enzymatic activation, or that can be deactivated by particular enzymes, may have their potency greatly affected by apparently innocuous agents that simply induce or inhibit the relevant enzymes in the target tissue. (For example, Wattenberg and Loub, 1978, suggested such a role for indoles in *Brassica* and other vegetables; *see also* Wattenberg, 1980, for a review of these and various other putative inhibitors of carcinogenesis.) Although innumerable instances will emerge where such mechanisms might theoretically be of relevance in humans, none have been demonstrated to be so. The most promising populations in which to seek such effects might be those where a single chemical carcinogen (e.g., aflatoxin in Mozambique) dominates the list of preventable causes of cancer, so only a few enzymes are of great importance.

3 (d) Deactivation or prevention of formation of short-lived intracellular active species.—Before they can damage the cells of the body, many carcinogens must be oxidized, yielding "metabolically activated" intermediates. (Indeed, most carcinogens detected by the Ames test, as described in section 4.2, are active only because the standard Ames test includes oxidative enzymes.) As well as "simple" addition of ordinary oxygen, in vivo mechanisms of oxidation and peroxidation include the generation of short-lived intermediates such as (i) oxidative free radicals or (ii) excited molecular oxygen. (For review, *see* the chapter by Foote, 1976, and the chapters that accompany it.) Consequently, the dangers from certain carcinogens might be reduced if appropriate parts of the body were

---

[29] Defined by the Analytical Methods Committee (1943) as the residue of carbohydrate food that resists extraction by boiling with 0.255 *N* sulfuric acid and subsequently with 0.313 *N* sodium hydroxide.

permeated with antioxidants, free radical traps, or quenchers of molecular excitation[30] (Ames et al., 1981).

(*i*) Free radicals: One of the chief intracellular systems (but not the only important one: Bize et al., 1980) for trapping *free radicals* and peroxides involves collaboration between vitamin E and a selenium-containing enzyme (which accounts, incidentally, for much of the selenium in people's bodies). Both selenium (as sodium selenide) and vitamin E can certainly protect laboratory animals against carcinogens under suitable experimental circumstances (Shamberger, 1970), although in other circumstances selenium may even enhance animal cancer onset rates; Griffin (1979) reviews both the dangers and the promise of selenium as a prophylactic against cancer. Selenium levels have been found by various authors to be lower in cancer patients than in controls, but until such studies are done prospectively, or in patients with tumors too small to disturb their appetite or general metabolism, this finding might as easily reflect the effects of the cancer on selenium as of selenium on carcinogenesis. Geographically, selenium intake varies widely from place to place within the United States and Canada, and inverse correlations with cancer risk have been reported (Schrauzer et al., 1976; Shamberger and Frost, 1969). But geographic correlations are, of course, not strong evidence for a true protective effect. High levels of selenium are, moreover, toxic, so its role should be evaluated with caution. Turning to vitamin E, clinical deficiency of it is so rare (and so easy to treat when diagnosed) that epidemiological study of vitamin E deficiency is difficult. However, people who habitually self-medicate with vitamin E or with multivitamin pills that contain vitamin E absorb from their gut more than ten times as much vitamin E as people who do not, and large prospective studies of cancer onset rates in relation to vitamin E self-medication have been started but are not yet informative. The potential importance of dietary selenium and vitamin E (and β-carotene, which can also trap free radicals: Packer et al., 1981) would justify considerably greater epidemiological efforts than have thus far been directed toward them.

(*ii*) Excited molecules: β-Carotene and various other carotenoids are also among the most efficient molecules discovered for quenching the energy of ("singlet") *excited oxygen*. β-Carotene is found in high concentration in carrots and in certain dark green leafy vegetables, and it and other carotenoids are also found in many other plant products in the American diet. β-Carotene is of nutritional interest as the precursor,

especially in poor countries, of much of the vitamin A in the normal human diet. (One molecule of β-carotene can be converted in the intestine into two molecules of vitamin A, although much of the β-carotene in the diet is absorbed directly from the gut and circulates unchanged around the body.) Perhaps because of this provitamin A activity, there have been many epidemiologic studies of the β-carotene levels in the blood or diet of cancer patients or of healthy people who subsequently develop cancer (for review, *see* Peto et al., 1981). Most such studies have indicated a reasonably consistent but not very extreme protective effect, and the results of the 20 available dietary studies are abstracted in table 13. These data are of interest for four reasons.

First, although the data in table 13 are consistent with the hypothesis that β-carotene has a protective effect, they clearly do not constitute strong evidence that it does so. The observed associations could easily have arisen merely because β-carotene intake is correlated with the intake of some truly protective (plant product?) component of diet or because β-carotene-containing vegetable intake is inversely correlated with some truly harmful (animal product?) component of diet. Further evidence should emerge from current studies of Brazilian populations where β-carotene is used heavily and regularly by some but not all of the population; but, even if β-carotene is really protective, sufficient evidence to justify advocacy of widespread dietary modification may not be obtainable except by long-term randomized intervention with β-carotene among apparently healthy people.

Second, the data in table 13 provide strong evidence that whether or not β-carotene itself is truly protective, some dietary factors that modify cancer risk are likely to exist; otherwise no material correlations, true or false, with β-carotene consumption should be evident. Moreover, since people already differ with respect to these factors, the factors should, once discovered, be modifiable in acceptable ways. (This may, however, be more true of insertion of protective agents into the diet than of removal of harmful factors from the diet.)

Third, even important real effects may not show up very clearly in epidemiologic studies of dietary factors. Let us imagine dividing the population into thirds with respect to their long-term average β-carotene intake, and let us for the moment suppose that, because of their lack of β-carotene, the bottom third have double the total cancer risk of the top third. Supplementing the diet of the bottom two groups with enough β-carotene to raise their intake to the level of the top group would then eliminate one-third of the total cancer rate, a hypothetical effect equivalent to that of abolishing tobacco! If real, such an effect would be of great importance, yet, due to the classification errors that would inevitably arise in the assessment of people's relative β-carotene intake by questionnaire, correlations no larger than those seen taking table 13 as a whole might be expected. This reemphasizes the need for unbiased randomized evaluation of such hypotheses whenever practicable.

---

[30] Short-lived oxidative intermediates include the hydroxyl radical OH·, the superoxide radical O_2^-·, and the singlet excited state $^1O_2$ of oxygen. Peroxides can be reduced by the Se-dependent enzyme glutathione peroxidase (GSH), and superoxides can be deactivated to oxygen by various enzymes, each dependent on a different trace element (Bize et al., 1980), the most important of which may be the Mn-dependent enzyme manganese superoxide dismutase (MnSOD).

TABLE 13.—*Results of 20 questionnaire studies[a,b] of cancer in populations subdivided by some estimate of "vitamin A" intake (chiefly in fact, in many of these studies, the β-carotene in certain vegetables)*

Country	Relative risks, (lower:higher dietary intake)	Cancers studied	
		No.	Type
Norway	2.6: 1	36	Lung[c]
	1.7: 1	228	Stomach[d]
	1.4: 1	278	Colorectal[d]
United States, Minnesota	1.5: 1	83	Stomach[d]
	1.4: 1	373	Colorectal[d]
United States, Buffalo, N.Y.	1.7: 1.5: 1	292	Lung[c]
	2.1: 1.9: 1.7: 1.2: 1.4: 1.2: 1	569	Bladder[c]
	1.9: 1.6: 1	122	Esophagus[c]
	3.0: 1.9: 2.1: 1	421	Larynx[c]
Singapore	2.2: 1	233	Lung[d]
United Kingdom	0.7:[e] 1.3: 1.4: 1.1: 1	104	Lung[c]
Israel	1.1: 1.1: 1	406	Gastrointestinal[f]
France	1.0: 1	200	Esophagus[f]
United Kingdom	1.7: 1.1: 1	514	Gastrointestinal[d]
United States: vegetarians	2.2: 0.9: 1	41	Colon[d]
Iran	1.7: 1	344	Esophagus[d]
Japan	1.3: 1	611	Lung, ♂[g]
	1.5: 1	196	Lung, ♀[g]
	2: 1	63	Prostate[g]
	1.15: 1	1,823	Stomach[g]

[a] Some of these studies were prospective and some were retrospective.
[b] For references, *see* Peto et al. (1981).
[c] Subdivision of individuals was based on a "vitamin A index," the major contributor to which is β-carotene.
[d] Subdivision based on a "vegetable index," including the major sources of β-carotene.
[e] Based on only 7 cancers.
[f] Subdivision based on a "β-carotene index."
[g] Subdivision based on a "frequency index" for vegetables that are carotene-rich (defined as >10 IU/g).

Fourth and finally, the β-carotene hypothesis underlines the need, for public health purposes, to identify causes rather than mechanisms. Even if, by means of a large, long-term, strictly randomized intervention study, β-carotene were proved to reduce cancer risks among apparently healthy people, this would still not be good evidence that the quenching of singlet oxygen is an important protective mechanism, for it is at least as plausible that β-carotene should act by virtue of being a precursor of vitamin A (albeit perhaps not in the gut), and it is also possible that it might act by some direct hormone-like mechanism, by affecting certain immune functions, or by trapping free radicals.

4. Affecting "Promotion" of Cells

4 (a) Vitamin A deficiency.—In experimental animals and in cell cultures, vitamin A (retinol) and its esters and analogs (retinoids) can reduce the probability that partially altered cells will become fully transformed and will successfully proliferate into a pathologic tumor, although in some experimental systems retinoids can have apparently opposite effects. In humans, two small studies (Kark et al., 1981; Wald et al., 1980a) of stored blood samples from apparently healthy people have both reported that among people of similar sex and age there is a significant inverse correlation between blood vitamin A levels and risk of subsequent cancer. This does not add up to proof of a cause-and-effect relationship and will not do so even if

confirmed by much larger studies, but it certainly suggests that circulating vitamin A *per se* protects against cancer. Consequently, if only the dietary or other factors that affect blood vitamin A were known, then these might offer a means of reducing cancer risks. Unfortunately, the body controls the level of vitamin A in the blood rather precisely by mechanisms that remain poorly understood (but seem chiefly hormonal). Except in frank vitamin A deficiency, which is rare in developed countries, the simple expedient of adding much more vitamin A than normal to the diet has little effect on the level of vitamin A in the blood, and so the observation that blood vitamin A levels are inversely correlated with cancer does not automatically suggest that dietary supplementation with vitamin A will materially affect cancer risks in developed countries such as the United States (Peto et al., 1981). It does, however, suggest that in poor countries a further consequence of chronic vitamin A deficiency may be an increased risk of cancer, especially since the normal source of vitamin A in poor countries is intestinal oxidation of β-carotene, a molecule that may alternatively reduce cancer risks in other ways.

4 (b) Retinol binding protein.—This protein seems to have no function other than to transport vitamin A (retinol) in the bloodstream, and it seems to be the chief avenue of control of blood vitamin A levels. Consequently, any factors that affect its rate of synthesis or degradation might affect blood vitamin A levels and, in turn, cancer risks. Estrogens are one of the few things known to affect blood vitamin A levels substantially in adequately nourished animals, and women who use oral contraceptives have elevated blood vitamin A levels. (We do not know whether postmenopausal hormone replacement therapy also affects blood vitamin A levels.) However (*see* section 5.9), there is little evidence for cancer avoidance (except perhaps of the ovary) resulting from oral contraceptives, while both postmenopausal and diet-derived estrogens may enhance the risk of endometrial cancer.

4 (c) Otherwise affecting stem cell differentiation.— The retinoids are of interest both in themselves and because they show that stem cell differentiation can be modified to an animal's advantage. Among dietary factors that might eventually be found to have important effects on stem cell differentiation, the three most promising (or, at least, fashionable!) categories seem to be protease inhibitors (which, if eaten, may diffuse throughout the body), hormonal factors (among which one should perhaps include retinol), and their endocrine determinants. Almost all hormonal factors could in principle be affected by diet and almost all could in principle affect the risk of one or another type of cancer, but such wide generalizations are of little interest until they can be supported by specific correlations in humans between effect and putative cause. (The particular case of diet-derived estrogens and endometrial cancer will be discussed below.) Turning to the phospholipids that comprise the outer walls of cells, their "profile" in terms of degree of saturation and exact chemical structure may have a large effect on the various prostaglandins of which they are precursors (which may in turn profoundly affect cellular behavior), and their "profile" is determined fairly directly by the exact nature of the components of dietary fat. The key to real progress in the study of dietary fat (as in the study of dietary fiber) may therefore be precise subdivision of the types of dietary fat and separate consideration of the particular subtypes (Carroll, 1980). Among hormonal factors, A. J. McMichael (personal communication) has emphasized the potential importance of those specifically secreted into the bloodstream by the cells of the digestive tract.

5. Overnutrition

5 (a), 5 (b), 5 (c) Variation of gross aspects of the diet of laboratory animals can have such profound effects on their risks of spontaneous or induced tumors that the role of overnutrition should perhaps come first rather than last on a list of aspects of diet which may affect the incidence of cancer, even though the relevant mechanisms remain obscure. The importance of gross aspects of nutrition was suggested 40 years ago by Tannenbaum's (1940) experiments on mice, which showed that restricting the intake of food without modifying the proportion of the individual constituents could halve the incidence of spontaneous tumors of the breast and lung and of a variety of cancers produced experimentally by known carcinogens. The underfed mice grew to one-half the size of those fully fed, but they were active and sleek, appeared perfectly healthy, and lived on average longer than the others. Since then, these and similar experiments have been repeated many times, and the protective effects of various types and degrees of dietary restrictions have been repeatedly demonstrated, sometimes with much more striking results than in Tannenbaum's original work. (For a list of striking examples, *see* Jose, 1979.) Roe and Tucker (1974), for example, randomized mice having a high spontaneous incidence of tumors between continuous ad libitum feeding, in which the mice chose to eat 6 grams of food per day in frequent small amounts, and intermittent feeding, in which every mouse was given 5 grams of food once per day, which was generally all eaten immediately. No clear difference in longevity ensued, but 32 non-fatal spontaneous tumors arose among the 40 continuously-fed mice while only 4 arose among the 40 intermittently-fed mice. (*See also* Tucker, 1979; Conybeare, 1980; and Roe, 1981.)

That Tannenbaum's experiments made little impact on cancer research is, perhaps, not surprising, because it would hardly be practicable to prescribe Tannenbaum's severe dietary restrictions for normal people, and we still have no clear idea of the mechanisms whereby dietary restriction protects laboratory animals. (More interest might have been aroused, however, if the freely fed mice had been described as obese instead of the mice on the restricted diet being described as small!)

That being overweight is associated to some degree with the risk of death from certain types of human cancer has long been suspected, and this has recently been confirmed (for several anatomic sites other than the lung) by the massive ACS study, to which we referred previously. The data obtained from observing 750,000 American men and women for 13 years (Lew and Garfinkel, 1979) are summarized in table 14. However, in view of the striking effects that nutritional factors can have on overall animal cancer rates, the association of obesity with the aggregate of all types of fatal human cancer is not particularly impressive. Indeed, although there is a consistent trend toward increasing total risk with increasing body weight among women, the trend among men is dominated by the irregular trend with respect to lung cancer, thin men and women having the greatest lung cancer risks.

These data are not likely to be biased by the effects of preexisting cancer on initial weight, because people who were sick, had a history of cancer, heart disease, or stroke, or had lost 10 pounds or more in weight over the preceding year were omitted from this analysis. Even so the results are not easy to interpret because weight is associated with a variety of social and behavioral characteristics not precisely standardized for and that affect the risk of cancer in other ways, including smoking habits and socioeconomic status (both, as it happens, inversely). The possibility also has to be considered that the diagnosis of cancer—and particularly cancer of the breast—may be delayed in the very obese, causing some increase in fatality. But

TABLE 14.—*Mortality ratios from various types of cancer, by weight index*[a]

Type of cancer	Patients' sex	Mortality ratio for weight index[b] in ranges:						
		<0.80 (Thin)	0.80– 0.89	0.90– 1.09	1.10– 1.19	1.20– 1.29	1.30– 1.39	≥1.40 (Large)
Endometrium	♀	0.89	1.04	1.00	1.36	1.85	2.30[d]	5.42
Gallbladder, plus biliary passages	♀	0.68[d]	0.74	1.00	1.59	1.74	1.80	3.58
Cervix	♀	0.76	0.77	1.00	1.24	1.51	1.42[d]	2.39
Kidney	♀	1.12	0.70	1.00	1.09	1.30	1.85	2.03[d]
Stomach	♂	1.34	0.61	1.00	1.22	0.97	0.73[d]	1.88[d]
	♀	0.74	0.95	1.00	1.07	1.28	1.26	1.03[d]
Colon, rectum	♂	0.90	0.86	1.00	1.26	1.23	1.53	1.73
	♀	0.93	0.84	1.00	0.96	1.10	1.30	1.22
Lymphoma	♀	0.83	1.14	1.00	1.06	1.00	0.92	1.13
Brain	♀	0.86	0.89	1.00	0.95	1.52	0.69[d]	1.01[d]
Leukemia	♀	0.73	1.00	1.00	1.01	0.88	0.85	1.24
Breast	♀	0.82	0.86	1.00	1.19	1.16	1.22	1.53
Prostate	♂	1.02	0.92	1.00	0.90	1.37	1.33	1.29[d]
Lung	♂	1.78	1.38	1.00	0.85	1.04	1.00	1.27
	♀	1.49	1.20	1.00	1.10	1.06	1.06	1.22
Ovary	♀	0.86	0.98	1.00	1.15	0.99	0.88	1.63
Pancreas	♂	1.20	0.82	1.00	0.91	0.88	0.76[d]	1.62[d]
	♀	1.17	1.06	1.00	1.36	1.43	1.18	0.61[d]
All cancers	♀	0.96	0.92	1.00	1.10	1.19	1.23	1.55
	♂	1.33	1.13	1.00	1.02	1.09	1.14	1.33

[a] Based on report by Lew and Garfinkel (1979) of data from ACS study of one million U.S. men and women during the 1960's. The tabulated mortality ratios, all of which are standardized for age and sex and a few crude categories of tobacco usage, compare cancer death rates with cancer death rate among people whose weight index[b] was 0.90–1.09.

[b] Actual weight divided by the average weight for people of similar height and sex. Values in the range 0.90–1.09 are close to average weight.

[c] Cancers were omitted for which some mortality ratios were based on <5 deaths.

[d] Ratio based on only 5–9 deaths.

even with these qualifications the ACS results, which are fully in accord with other clinical and epidemiological evidence, strongly suggest that those forms of overnutrition which lead to obesity may play a major part in the development of cancer of the endometrium and gallbladder in women and possibly a lesser part in causing several other types of cancer in both sexes.

It is easy to understand that overnutrition should be a major factor in the development of cancer of the endometrium (Armstrong, 1977), because the disease can be produced by excessive exposure to estrogen and the only natural estrogens to which women are exposed after the menopause are made from adrenal hormones in adipose tissue. After the menopause, the level of estrogens in the blood (if they are not prescribed medically) is directly proportional to the degree of adiposity. Apart from cancer of the endometrium, no other type of cancer has been related so definitely to overnutrition or to a specific component of the common American or European diet, except insofar as a high standard of nutrition in childhood also advances the age at menarche, which, in view of the association that exists between early menarche and breast cancer risk, will presumably increase the subsequent risk of breast cancer. There are, however, several findings that encourage the belief that the incidence of many of the common types of cancer is determined in large part by individual components of diet or by their general balance.

For example, colorectal and breast cancer are generally associated with a high standard of living in adult life and have been suspected of being due to diets containing a high proportion of fat or possibly (in the case of colorectal cancer) of meat. Correlations (text-fig. 1 on page 1205) between the national consumption of fat and meat per head of population and the incidence of these types of cancer are strong (Armstrong and Doll, 1975a)—nearly as strong as the correlation between the consumption of fat and the incidence of endometrial cancer. However, these cancers are not uniformly uncommon in vegetarians, and the low incidence in Seventh-day Adventists (who are largely vegetarian) is matched by a similarly low incidence in Mormons (who are not vegetarians and who do not avoid fat in their diet) (West et al., 1980; Lyon et al., 1980; Phillips et al., 1980; Enstrom, 1980). Gaskill et al. (1979) have pointed out that the mortality from breast cancer within different national and racial groups correlates with the proportion of the population that continues in adult life to secrete substantial amounts of lactase (an enzyme produced to aid the digestion of milk), and they find that within the United States breast cancer mortality correlates more strongly with the consumption of milk fat than of other types of fat. This offers an interesting line for further inquiry, but for the time being the real reasons for the strong international correlations in text-figure 1 must still be considered obscure.

Conclusion

Our discussion of the ways and means whereby dietary factors may importantly affect cancer onset rates has inevitably omitted many interesting possibilities. Particularly, some of the many vitamins, trace elements, other micronutrients, enzyme inducers, and protease inhibitors that we have not mentioned could be important, as may the particular subtypes of fat, fiber, and digestible carbohydrates that we have not discussed in separate detail. This is not to say that everything is important; when more is understood, a few factors will presumably be of much greater importance than the many others, and the ultimate aim of research must be to identify reliably these few important modifiable factors. Three general points are suggested by our review. First, even though dietary intake of powerful carcinogens or precarcinogens as components of natural, stored, or cooked foods may not be an avoidable cause of a large proportion of U.S. cancers, dietary factors may influence cancer risks in a variety of indirect ways. Second, among these indirect ways, both enhancing and protective mechanisms may be discovered. But, since prescription of dietary additives may prove more acceptable than proscription of harmful dietary habits, any protective mechanisms may be of more immediate public health significance. Third, the role of laboratory research and observational epidemiologic research should perhaps be seen as generation of about a dozen "most promising" hypotheses. Although any single one of these may be more likely to be false than true, it is more likely than not that at least one or two of these dozen hypotheses will be true and really important. It may be that for some particular dietary hypothesis observational epidemiological evidence of its truth will be adduced that is as wholly convincing as the epidemiological evidence proving beyond reasonable doubt that cigarette smoking causes lung cancer. For most dietary factors, however, even if they are among the few really important truly causal or truly protective factors, such clear-cut evidence may not be possible either from epidemiological observations or from laboratory studies. These will be the chief methods by which the "top twelve" hypotheses are devised, but they may not be the methods whereby these hypotheses can be tested, particularly because (even despite the interestingly bizarre behavior of many people!) it may be impossible to find two reasonably similar populations whose diet has differed for decades only in the one factor of interest. Consequently, wherever this is practicable, apparently promising hypotheses should be tested rigorously by randomized intervention in large populations.

The number of people that putatively preventive measures may be relevant to is so large that the methodological rigor appropriate for determining what really prevents cancer should, if anything, be greater than for evaluating cancer therapy, and not (as now) much less. There is no reason for large intervention trials to be impracticable or to be as expensive as they have been in vascular disease. Any of the putatively protective non-toxic vitamins, trace elements, micro-nutrients, protease inhibitors, or antioxidants that finish up in the top twelve hypotheses might be thus testable, as might intake of various putatively protective types of fat or fiber. If several[31] such randomized interventions are undertaken (in the expectation that only one or two should work), progress toward reliable knowledge of what is really important may be greatly accelerated.

The outcome of future controlled laboratory research and of the epidemiologic observation of human risks may well be, in our view, that diet will be shown to be a factor in determining the occurrence of a high proportion of all cancers of the stomach and large bowel as well as of the body of the uterus (endometrium), gallbladder, and (in tropical countries) of the liver. Diet may also prove to have a material effect on the incidence of cancers of the breast and pancreas and, perhaps through the anti-carcinogenic effects of various micronutrients, on the incidence of cancers in many other tissues. If this is so, it may be possible to reduce U.S. cancer death rates by practicable dietary means by as much as 35% ("guestimated" as stomach and large bowel, 90%; endometrium, gallbladder, pancreas, and breast, 50%; lung, larynx, bladder, cervix, mouth, pharynx, and esophagus, 20%; other types of cancer, 10%). Although this figure of 35% is a plausible total, the parts that contribute to it are uncertain in the extreme, so the degree of uncertainty of the total should be obvious, and we make no pretense of its reliability. It is still possible (though rather unlikely) that no practicable modifications of diet will be discovered that can reduce total U.S. cancer death rates by more than 10%, but it is equally possible that reductions of perhaps even double our suggested total of 35% might ultimately be achievable, although this certainly cannot be expected in the near future.

5.4 Food Additives

Chemicals are added to food to preserve it and to give it color, flavor, and consistency. Preservation of food is essential in modern society because food is grown in one part of the world and consumed in another part weeks, months, or even years later. The justification for the addition of chemicals to food to give it color, flavor, and consistency is less obvious but not always altogether negligible. Artificial sweeteners, for example, help some people consume less sugar and so (perhaps) avoid undesirable obesity. With rare exceptions, the individual consumer has no useful knowledge of what chemicals are consumed, and it may be extremely difficult for the consumer to obtain any

---

[31] More than one intervention could be evaluated in a single such trial by the use of "factorial trial" designs (Peto, 1978). Note that, because of the typical delay of decades between initiation and cancer onset, it is practicable to evaluate randomly only factors that affect the *later* stages of neoplastic transformation.

direct evidence of their effect on humans. Food additives have therefore been subject to extremely careful laboratory screening before they are used. Some definitely carcinogenic chemicals were used for a time before their carcinogenicity in animals was discovered and have now been withdrawn. These included butter yellow (DAB), thiourea, and (in Japan only) the food preservative AF2. Whether they have produced appreciable numbers of cancers in humans is unknown. Of the many additives now used, three require special consideration: (i) saccharin, (ii) butylated hydroxytoluene, and (iii) nitrites.

(i) Saccharin.—This has been shown to cause cancer of the bladder in rats (more clearly in males than in females) in two circumstance: 1) when given in straightforward feeding studies, especially when given over two generations and 2) when given after a single instillation into the bladder of a powerful carcinogen (N-methyl-N-nitrosourea). In both cases the quantities of saccharin that had to be given were large (constituting a few percent of the feed). No convincing evidence has been obtained of the production of cancer in other organs nor in other animals (mice, hamsters, and monkeys), but many of these experiments have involved only small numbers of animals and have been, in other ways, imperfect (Office of Technology Assessment, 1977). Three short-term tests have produced evidence of activity (including the production of sister chromatid exchange), whereas seven others (including the standard Ames test and a test for the transformation of mammalian cells) have not (Office of Technology Assessment, 1977).

In sum, there is no doubt that saccharin (even without the small proportion of impurities that are always present in the commercial preparations) is capable of causing cancer in defined conditions, but its mechanisms of action are obscure and it is certainly not a powerful animal carcinogen. It is therefore a matter of judgment, on which opinions may reasonably differ, what effects doses between two and three orders of magnitude lower (in mg/kg/day) are likely to have on humans. The human evidence collected over the last few years fails to distinguish clearly between saccharin and cyclamates, but it is more relevant to the former as the use of saccharin began earlier (in 1902) and has continued longer. First, but very crudely, there is no suggestion of an increase in the mortality from bladder cancer that could be attributed to the introduction of saccharin (Armstrong and Doll, 1974). Second, diabetics, who use more saccharin than do most other people, tend to have a lower, rather than a higher, incidence of the disease (Kessler, 1970; Armstrong and Doll, 1975b; Armstrong et al., 1976). This should not be interpreted to mean that saccharin prevents cancer but may be explained either by some physiological effect of diabetes or, more probably, by a tendency for diabetics to smoke less heavily than average (perhaps because many of the diabetics who do smoke are killed by heart disease before they reach old age). Third, case-control studies show almost identical use of artificial sweeteners by individuals, irrespective of whether they have developed bladder cancer or not.

The overall results of the five largest and best controlled studies are summarized in table 15. One of the estimated relative risks for male users of saccharin is just statistically significant, but the rest range neatly on either side of 1.0. Division of the patients into groups by amount and duration of use and adjustment to allow for the effects on bladder cancer of cigarette smoking and of occupation (both of which effects are demonstrated by all the studies that examined them) provides no evidence of a consistent biological relationship with saccharin. As would be expected if saccharin were irrelevant to bladder cancer, in some subgroups of certain studies apparently positive relationships between saccharin and disease appear, while in other subgroups of those studies negative relationships appear, and the sum of the human evidence could hardly be more null, at least for cancer of the bladder, which was the anatomic site affected by saccharin in rats. Equally careful studies of saccharin use in relation to other types of human cancer are not available, but the lack of any unexpected excesses of any type of cancer among diabetics is moderately reassuring.

Disparity between the results of tests in different animal species is common, and the apparent disparity between some animal and in vitro tests and the human evidence is no cause for surprise. However, human exposure to a weak carcinogen may need to be prolonged for several decades before any positive effect can be detected, and no assurance can be given that an effect will not be produced by a lifetime of exposure to the unusually large amounts that are consumed in diet drinks by some children and young adults. For our present purpose, however, we can conclude that the

TABLE 15.—*Risk of bladder cancer with use of artificial sweeteners*

Authors	Patients		Relative risk with use of:		
	No.	Sex	Table-top sweeteners	Diet beverages	Artificial sweeteners, any form
Howe et al. (1977)	408	♂	1.6	0.8	—
Kessler and Clark (1978)	365	♂	0.88	0.95	0.97
			—	—	1.08[a]
Hoover et al. (1980)	2,226	♂	1.04	0.95	0.99
Morrison and Buring (1980)	469	♂	0.8	0.8	
Wynder and Stellman (1980)	302	♂	0.93	0.85	—
Howe et al. (1977)	152	♀	0.6	0.9	—
Kessler and Clark (1978)	154	♀	0.91	1.00	1.00
			—	—	0.87[a]
Hoover et al. (1980)	744	♀	1.04	0.97	1.01
Morrison and Buring (1980)	197	♀	1.5	1.6	—
Wynder and Stellman (1980)	65	♀	0.62	0.60	—

[a] Specifically saccharin.

proportion of human bladder cancers now attributable to the use of artificial sweeteners is negligible.

(ii) Butylated hydroxytoluene.—This has been used extensively as an antioxidant for many years. It is not carcinogenic by itself, but it has been reported to enhance the production of lung tumors by urethan in mice (Witschi et al., 1977). Conversely, its antioxidant effect has been found to inhibit the formation of active carcinogens in the laboratory (Wattenberg, 1978), and a similar effect might be expected to occur in vivo. Conceivably, its use—and perhaps that of the more common butylated hydroxyanisole—has contributed to the decline in mortality from stomach cancer, but no reliable human evidence for or against this hypothesis is known to us.

(iii) Nitrites.—These have been used to preserve meat since the last century and have already been discussed in company with the natural components of food in section 5.3. According to Shubik (1980), the nitrite added to food constitutes only 10% of the total nitrite reaching the stomach in vegetables and saliva. If, however, the formation of nitrosamines and nitros- amides in the intestinal tract proves to be of practical importance, dietary nitrite, of which nitrite used as a food additive is a part, must be held responsible for some cases of cancer. Nitrite used as a food additive may, moreover, be disproportionately important because it reaches the stomach in concentrated packets and reacts chemically in proportion to the square of its concentration. The National Research Council's (1978) Panel on Nitrates was unable to reach any conclusions about the quantitative effect of nitrates, but the council advised that reasonable measures be taken to minimize human exposure to N-nitroso compounds, including the restriction of the amounts of nitrate and nitrite added to meat products.

Because of the uncertainty regarding the position of nitrites and the possibility that other additives might have unsuspected effects, we have not excluded food additives as a source of risk but have attributed to them a token proportion of less than 1%.

5.5 Reproductive and Sexual Behavior

Changes in the body resulting from sexual inter- course, pregnancy, childbirth, and lactation are in a different class from those produced by exposure to chemicals in the ambient atmosphere. They are, how- ever, environmental in origin, insofar as they are not solely the product of the individual's own genetic material, and they were certainly regarded as "extrinsic factors" by the WHO (1964) expert committee on the prevention of cancer, which defined extrinsic factors as including "modifying factors" that favor neoplasia of apparently intrinsic origin (e.g., hormone imbalances). The impact of these factors varies greatly from com- munity to community, and study of the way the processes of reproduction affect the incidence of cancer may well throw light on the mechanism of carcino- genesis in the relevant organs, perhaps indicating ways

(short of encouraging or discouraging reproduction!) in which an important group of cancers can be prevented.

The most obvious relationship is that observed between sexual intercourse and the development of cancer of the cervix uteri. This disease occurs in virgins, but only with extreme rarity. It is more common in women who have had several children than in women who have had only one, and it was for a long time thought to be due to the trauma of childbirth. Now, however, it appears that the number of children is not directly relevant and that the risk of developing the disease is chiefly related to the number of sexual partners. Whether the risk for women who have had only one sexual partner is also increased if that partner had previously had multiple partners remains to be proved, but the present evidence strongly suggests that one of the primary causes of the disease is an agent passed between partners in intercourse, quite possibly a virus. If this is indeed so, it may eventually be possible to protect against the disease by immunization, by treatment of the infection, by closer attention to personal hygiene, or by the use of obstructive methods of contraception. Meanwhile, of course, the impact of the disease can be greatly reduced by regular vaginal examination and the treatment of women in whom a smear shows evidence of pre-malignant change.

Pregnancy and childbirth, for their part, seem to play a significant role in the prevention of cancers of the endometrium, ovary, and breast, all these condi- tions being somewhat less common in women who have borne children early than in women who have had no children. The relationship with cancer of the breast, which has been reviewed by MacMahon et al. (1973), is particularly striking, breast cancer in parous women becoming progressively less likely to develop as the age of first pregnancy decreases. A pregnancy leading to abortion does not have the same protective effect as one that goes to term, and it is probable that the effect is produced by the first stimulus to lactation which somehow diminishes the risk of the subsequent initiation of a cancer. Lactation itself, however, seems to have no material effect, irrespective of whether it is suppressed or prolonged. Finally, the risk of cancer of the breast is diminished by a late onset of menstruation (made more likely by undernutrition) and by an early menopause.

Cancer of the cervix currently accounts for some 1.5% of all U.S. cancer deaths, but the number is decreasing due at least in part to the more widespread use of cervical screening and to the increasing proportion of women who, having had a hysterectomy some time previously, have no uterus and so no risk of uterine cancer. Comparison of the total number of deaths from cancer of the uterine cervix with the small number that would have been expected if the low rates typical of nuns had prevailed throughout the United States suggests that the large majority of cases of cancer of the uterine cervix are due to the (presumably infective) processes reviewed above, prevention or treatment of which might, therefore, reduce total cancer mortality by 1%.

It is not clear how far it will be possible to reduce the incidence rates of cancers of the breast, ovary, and endometrium (which together account for 29% of all U.S. female cancer deaths) when we understand the mechanisms whereby reproductive factors influence them. It is difficult to believe that no preventive strategies will be discovered for these cancers, since reproductive activity affects them so profoundly. Whether practicable preventive strategies will emerge within the next decade or two is, however, so uncertain that neither pessimism nor optimism can yet be refuted. These cancers collectively account for 13% of all U.S. cancer deaths, and estimates of the percentage that will be avoidable by mechanisms related to the mechanisms whereby reproduction exerts its effects might range between 0 and 12%. We have arbitrarily taken a middle figure of 6% and have added to it the definite 1% of deaths that would be avoidable by control of the causes of cervical cancer, to get an estimate of 7% thus avoidable. Note, however, that reproductive and dietary factors might well interact multiplicatively (*see* section 4.4) in the production of these cancers, unless diet affects them by a hormonal mechanism, and in either situation, this estimate of 7% and the percentage preventable by dietary modification will overlap.

5.6 Occupation

The observation that led to the discovery of the first pure chemical carcinogen and a year later to the isolation of the powerful carcinogen benzo[a]pyrene from a natural product (Cook et al., 1932, 1933) derived directly from the observation of a British surgeon at the end of the 18th century that cancer of the scrotum occurred characteristically in people who had been chimney sweeps in whom, to quote his words, "the disease . . . seems to derive from a lodgment of soot in the rugae [folds] of the scrotum" (Pott, 1775). In the years that followed Pott's observation, many other groups of workers have been found to suffer from specific hazards of cancer. The search for such occupational hazards (some affecting large and some affecting small groups of workers) has unearthed more substances known to cause cancer in humans than any other method has done.

That this should be so is not surprising, as industrial chemicals have been used freely in the past unless a few simple tests on animals or a brief experience of

TABLE 16.—*Established occupational causes of cancer* (*See also Table 6*)

Agent	Site of cancer	Occupation[a]
Aromatic amines (4-aminodiphenyl, benzidine, 2-naphthylamine)	Bladder	Dye manufacturers, rubber workers, coal gas manufacturers
Arsenic[b]	Skin, lung	Copper and cobalt smelters, arsenical pesticide manufacturers, some gold miners
Asbestos	Lung, pleura, peritoneum (also probably[c] stomach, large bowel, esophagus)	Asbestos miners, asbestos textile manufacturers, asbestos insulation workers, certain shipyard workers
Benzene	Marrow, especially erythroleukemia	Workers with glues and varnishes
Bischloromethyl ether	Lung	Makers of ion-exchange resins
Cadmium[b]	Prostate	Cadmium workers
Chromium[b]	Lung	Manufacturers of chromates from chrome ore, pigment manufacturers
Ionizing radiations	Lung	Uranium and some other miners
Ionizing radiations	Bone	Luminizers
Ionizing radiations	Marrow, all sites	Radiologists, radiographers
Isopropyl oil	Nasal sinuses	Isopropyl alcohol manufacturers
Mustard gas	Larynx, lung	Poison gas manufacturers
Nickel[b]	Nasal sinuses, lung	Nickel refiners
Polycyclic hydrocarbons in soot, tar, oil	Skin, scrotum, lung	Coal gas manufacturers, roofers, asphalters, aluminum refiners, many groups selectively exposed to certain tars and oils
UV light	Skin	Farmers, seamen
Vinyl chloride	Liver (angiosarcoma)	PVC manufacturers
—[d]	Nasal sinuses	Hardwood furniture manufacturers
—[d]	Nasal sinuses	Leather workers

[a] Typical occupations in which exposure to the listed agents has been proved to confer a hazard of cancer of one or more of these sites. (Some of these broad occupational categories also include, of course, many people who have never worked with the listed agents.)
[b] Certain compounds or oxidation states only.
[c] Studies of American asbestos workers have reported a significant excess of deaths certified as being due to cancers of the digestive tract, but various studies elsewhere have not. Although probably real (rather than representing miscertified mesotheliomas or respiratory tract cancers), there is not yet general agreement on this point [Acheson (1980)].
[d] Causative agent not known.

their use had shown them to be acutely poisonous. Table 16 lists the substances that have been shown by epidemiology to be carcinogenic, the occupational carcinogens that were first shown to be carcinogenic in the laboratory, and the occupations that are known to produce a risk of cancer even though the specific substances responsible have not yet been identified. The hazards that have been recognized thus far tend to be those which increase the relative risk of some particular type(s) of cancer very substantially, and important occupational hazards may quite possibly exist that have not yet been detected because the added risk is small compared with that due to other causes, or because only a few people have been exposed, or simply because a hazard has not been suspected and so not looked for. It must also be borne in mind that cancer in humans seldom develops until one or more decades after beginning exposure to a carcinogen, and it is too soon to be sure whether agents are human carcinogens if they were introduced into industry only during the last 20 years. Consequently, we do not yet know whether the decrease of certain occupations over the past quarter century and the increase in others will on balance increase or decrease the number of occupational cancers arising at around the end of the century, nor do we know what the net effects by then will be of the discontinuation of use of a few chemicals and of the introduction of many more, sometimes on an enormous scale (text-fig. 8; however, increases in plant automation and allied practices may mean *less* total worker exposure now than in earlier years for some but not for all major products, at least during primary manufacture).

Total Effects of Occupational Factors: Limitations of Current Data

On present knowledge, therefore, it is impossible to make any precise estimate of the proportion of the cancers of today that are attributable to hazards at work (let alone how many future cancers may arise from past occupational exposure during the years before 1980), and none of the estimates that have been made are claimed to be anything more than informed guesses. It is, therefore, odd that despite the passionate debates that have taken place about the likely magnitude of the number of U.S. cancer deaths that are or will be attributable to occupation, no routine system has been adopted in the United States for generating reliable information. The efforts of Milham (1976) in Washington State to relate the certified cause of death to the crude information about occupation that should be recorded on all death certificates have pointed to some real industrial hazards, and this inexpensive but demonstrably practical method of screening for gross hazards could be extended to many other States in the United States, although it might overlook some widespread but moderate hazards. Information on particular occupations or factories could be obtained either by routinely monitoring, perhaps by the newly established National Death Index, cancer mortality among all past

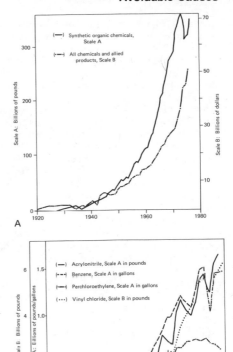

TEXT-FIGURE 8.—Examples of the rapidity of the growth of the industrial production of certain chemicals during the mid-20th century (Davis and Magee, 1979; reprinted with permission of *Science* and D. L. Davis).
A) *Annual production of chemicals as a whole, 1920–present (excludes tar and primary products from petroleum and natural gas).*
B) *Annual production of four animal or human carcinogens.*

and present employees of particular factories (from employers' and/or union records where possible, since Social Security and Internal Revenue Service records may be unavailable[32] or imprecise). Information on the totality of cancer could in principle be obtained by establishing an ongoing case–control study (*see* below) of a representative sample of all cancer cases (weighted

---

[32] Restrictions exist on the transfer of information on where people have been employed from the Internal Revenue Service to research workers in NIOSH and other parts of the National Institutes of Health. These restrictions make it unnecessarily difficult to determine which occupations may affect the health of the workers who pursue them, and we would strongly endorse the recommendation (Subcommittee on Oversight and Investigations, 1980) that they be relaxed. We know of no instance in any country in the world where the provision of information for epidemiological research has led to any abuse of privacy and many instances where the lack of such information has led to unnecessary disease.

perhaps in favor of cancer in younger adults and of cancers of the bladder and respiratory tract in persons of all ages) in relation to occupation and smoking, but since the chief uncertainty in the effects of occupational factors relates (see below) to cancer of the lung, such a study should in practice be restricted chiefly or wholly to this disease.

In the absence of direct information from a nationally representative case-control study such as this, the most usual approach has been to consider separately each type of cancer, to attribute a proportion of each type of cancer to occupation on the basis of a few geographically restricted case-control studies, or, in the complete absence of any such data, on the basis of clinical impressions and then to combine the figures in proportion to the frequency with which each type of cancer occurs. Perhaps use of such methods led Higginson (1979), Higginson and Muir (1977 and 1979), and Wynder and Gori (1977) to suggest figures of less than 5% for the percentage of all cases of cancer due to occupational hazards and Cole (1977) to suggest a figure less than 10%. In no case, however, were the methods used characterized, so detailed criticism of these estimates is impossible.

The "OSHA" Paper (NCI/NIEHS/NIOSH) of 1978

More recently, another approach has been used in a paper "contributed to" by 10 research workers of the National Cancer Institute, the National Institute of Environmental Health Sciences, and the National Institute for Occupational Safety and Health. (It is sometimes referred to as "Bridbord et al., 1978," but in ignorance of the responsible author(s) we shall refer to it subsequently as the "OSHA paper," as it was filed at the Occupational Safety and Health Administration in a post-hearing record on September 15, 1978.) It has been widely cited from the moment in 1978 when Mr. Califano, then Secretary of Health, Education, and Welfare, publicly accepted its conclusions. In it, an attempt was made to calculate the proportion of cancers attributable to occupation using quantitative estimates of the effects of six known carcinogens and of the numbers of workers exposed to them, which led to the conclusion (OSHA, 1978) that

> Reasonable projections of the future consequences of past exposure to established carcinogens suggest that . . . occupationally related cancers may comprise as much as 20% or more of total cancer mortality. Asbestos alone will probably contribute up to 13–18%, and the data (relating to five other carcinogens) suggest at least 10–20% more.

Added together, this makes 23–38% of the total, to which we would still have to add the effects of ionizing radiations, other known carcinogens excluded from the calculations, and other occupational hazards that have not yet been detected but which, in all probability, exist.

If these estimates were reliable, it would be extremely encouraging, in the sense that they would indicate a simple way in which a large proportion of all cancers could be prevented. We have, therefore, examined the calculations that led to these estimates in detail (see appendix F). They involve three main steps.

First, the proportion of cancer deaths that are, or will be over the next few decades, caused by ever having been employed (in or before the 1970's) in industries which use asbestos was estimated to be 13–18%, a figure substantially higher than that proposed by certain other commentators (e.g., Hogan and Hoel, 1981, from the National Institute of Environmental Health Sciences).

Second, six "established" industrial carcinogens were considered, one being asbestos, and projected numbers were estimated of excess cases of cancer to be expected in the future among people currently (1972/4) employed in industries using those six agents.

Third, it was noted that the total cancer risks projected for current employees in the other five of these six industries was if anything greater than the total projected for current employees in asbestos-using industries.[33] Since the proportion of cancer deaths that are, or will be over the next few decades, due to ever-exposure to asbestos had already been estimated as 13–18%, it was assumed without formal explanation that the proportion due to ever-exposure to the other five agents should be "at least 10% to 20%" (i.e., about double[34] the total risk projected for current exposure to these five agents). Simple addition then yielded a total of 23–38%, to which it was suggested the effects of many other occupational carcinogens must also be added.

This third part of the OSHA argument obviously depended on the at least approximate validity of the estimates of total risk in the first and second part of it. However, these estimates of total risk were so grossly in error that no arguments based even loosely on them should be taken seriously. The method used for projection of the future annual risks among current employees in each of the six industries was to multiply the number of millions of workers currently employed there, irrespective of their actual duration or degree of exposure (which will be negligible in many cases), by the percentage excess risks of cancer that have been observed by special epidemiological study in the United States or elsewhere among a few hundred or a few thousand workers who have been heavily exposed for many years to the agent of interest. This disregard of both dose and duration of exposure is indefensible and produces risk estimates which are more than ten times

---

[33] Actually, the former was more than double the latter.

[34] The suggestion elsewhere in the OSHA document that the total risk among current employees should be multiplied by a factor of "4–5" to allow for the fact that there may be four or five times as many ever-employees as current employees was not implemented; otherwise, the proportion due to ever-exposure to the other five agents would have been about 30%, and twice as many lung cancers as currently occur in the whole United States would have been ascribed to these six particular agents alone.

too large (appendix F). The error involved is quite as gross as to suppose that a non-smoker who works in a factory where other people smoke cigarettes will have a 20% risk of lung cancer because he is passively exposed to some cigarette smoke and 20% of heavy cigarette smokers get lung cancer.

In the first part of the OSHA paper, a similarly defective method was applied to the estimation of the total (lifelong) hazard to be expected among the 8-11 million or so living or dead Americans with some history of industrial exposure to asbestos. These are divided into 4 million "heavily exposed," 1.25 or 1.6 million (see appendix F) of whom are to be killed by asbestos, and 4-7 million "less heavily exposed," 0.4-0.7 million of whom are to be killed by asbestos. There is no reason to accept either of these sets of risk estimates, and there is good evidence that in total they are at least ten times too large (appendix F).

It seems likely that whoever wrote the OSHA paper (it has a list of "contributors," but no listed authors) did so for political rather than scientific purposes, and it will undoubtedly continue in the future as in the past to be used for political purposes by those who wish to emphasize the importance of occupational factors, including the Toxic Substances Strategy Committee in their 1980 report to the U.S. President as well as many newspaper articles and much scientific journalism. However, although its conclusions continue to be widely cited the crucial parts of the arguments for these conclusions have, perhaps advisedly, never been published in a scientific journal nor in any of the regular series of government publications. Unless they are, with proper attribution of responsible authorship, we would suggest that the OSHA paper should not be regarded as a serious contribution to scientific thought and should not be cited or used as if it were. (Furthermore, any suggestions which derive directly or indirectly from it that 20, 23, 38, or 40% of cancer deaths are, or will be, due to occupational factors should be dismissed.)

If estimates of the current proportion of cancers attributable to occupational factors are to be made, it seems unwise to try to make them by estimating the number of workers that have been exposed to some agent and "estimating" their excess relative risk of cancer. Even if deliberate bias is avoided (as, for example, by Hogan and Hoel, 1981, for asbestos), the data bearing on the likely magnitude of the excess risk are in most instances so unreliable (especially for the large numbers of less heavily exposed people) that substantial errors are probable, unless the estimate of relative risk derives from direct epidemiological observation of a strictly representative random sample of the workers to whose future it will be applied.

Practical Studies That Would Estimate Reliably the Current Effects of Occupational Factors

We do not, ourselves, consider particularly reliable any explicit numerical estimates of the proportion of cancers currently ascribable to occupation, since although the available data do indicate the order of magnitude of this proportion (see below), they do not permit its direct estimation. Data could, however, be collected in the course of only 2 or 3 years that would lead to a reasonably reliable estimate if a case–control study were commissioned comparable to but on a larger scale than that recently done by Hoover et al. (1980) for the National Cancer Institute which examined the possibility of a relationship between cancer of the bladder and the consumption of saccharin. (Although the case–control study by Williams et al., 1977, of occupational factors may seem to have been on a larger scale inasmuch as 7,518 patients were interviewed, fewer than one-tenth of these had cancer of the lung.)

Any such study of lung cancer should attempt to record occupational histories in as much detail as memory and knowledge of the processes on which the subject worked will permit; this would facilitate estimation of which agents or circumstances people have actually been exposed to. For discussion of theoretical and practical details, see Siemiatycki et al., 1981; perhaps surprisingly, the total costs of a typical case-control study are not increased by a large percentage, even if the length of the interview is doubled. However, although there is considerable merit in the suggestion by Siemiatycki et al., 1981, that patients with non-respiratory cancer could serve as "controls" for lung cancer patients (and vice versa), some cancer-free controls should also be included if the total effects of occupational factors are to be assessed convincingly. Also, of course, fine attention to the detail of individual case histories must not divert attention from the absolute requirement that large numbers of cases be studied.

Detailed occupational histories would have to be taken from 10,000 or so patients suffering from lung cancer (plus, if the contribution of occupation to other cancers is to be assessed, at least as many patients suffering from other selected cancers), and a comparable number of other men and women not affected by cancer would serve as controls. If, as we hope, the recent study by Hoover et al. (1980) proves to have adequate information on bladder cancer, it would not be necessary to include a further sample of patients with cancer of this particular type. Further inquiries would then have to be focused on the industries and occupations that were reported more often in the histories given by the cancer patients than in those reported by the control subjects. Many of these industries and occupations would have been reported more often by chance alone, and a second inquiry might be needed to see which of them were reported more frequently by the cancer patients on each occasion (although the use of James–Stein estimators may help avoid some of the statistical pitfalls in the testing of multiple data-derived hypotheses; Efron and Morris, 1977, discuss the principles involved). Consideration must then be given to the possibility that men and women engaged in the occupations reported more often by the cancer patients might tend to have other personal characteristics that affect the risk of cancer. Two characteristics in particular must be taken into account: smoking habits and socioeconomic status. The first has become of major importance as the prevalence of cigarette smoking varies with a host of social factors, ranging from education to alcoholism, some of which might determine (or be determined by) a person's occupation. It must, therefore, be expected that the incidence of lung cancer will tend to be higher in people employed in occupations in which the prevalence of cigarette smoking, and particularly long-term cigarette smoking, is high. The second, socioeconomic status, has long been known to be a major determinant of the incidence of cancers of the stomach and cervix uteri, which have consistently been found to be higher in unskilled and heavy manual workers (or their wives) irrespective of the nature of their occupation, than in more skilled manual workers, clerical workers, and men and women occupied in professions.

The importance of taking into account the general socioeconomic factors that affect the incidence of cancer across a wide range of occupations is illustrated by Fox and Adelstein's (1978) analysis of the occupational mortality statistics reported by the Registrar General for England and Wales (1978) for 1970–72. Standardization for "socioeconomic class" of the mortality ratios for cancer in 25 main occupational orders suggested that some 88% of the total variation could be accounted for by social differences of one sort or another. This estimate is, of course, extremely crude and is affected by many factors that may exaggerate or reduce the residual differences among occupations, but it provides a warning against incautious interpretation of differences in the risks of lung cancer seen in different occupations (as in Menck and Henderson, 1976). One

factor that Fox and Adelstein (1978) could allow for in part was smoking habits. They knew, from the results of the British General Household Survey (1978), that the proportion of men who smoked in each of the 25 occupational orders varied from 65% to over 130% of the national average, and they were able to show that these 25 percentages correlated fairly closely with the corresponding mortality ratios for cancer of the lung (text-fig. 9). They were not, however, able to allow for other important aspects of the smoking habit. (For example, Wynder, by personal communication, reports higher than average mean tar levels among the cigarettes smoked by blue-collar workers.)

Finally, special inquiries would have to be made to see whether the risk of cancer varied with the length and intensity of exposure to any specific environmental features of the occupations that had been picked out by the above methods.

Stop-Gap Methods of Estimating the Approximate Current Effects of Occupation

Until objective, nationally representative studies are undertaken, a more realistic assessment of the role of occupational hazards can probably be obtained by considering each type of cancer separately and estimating for each type the possible contribution of occupation. This may be a more reliable procedure in our present state of ignorance than trying to make a quantitative estimate of the hazards associated with broad groups of occupations without any reliable knowledge of the quantity of carcinogens to which men and women employed in them were actually exposed. We will, therefore, use our preferred method, realizing that those who disagree with our interpreta-

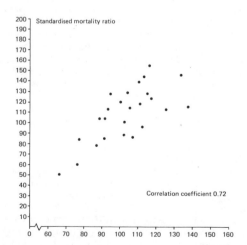

Order		Lung cancer SMR	Smoking score*
I	Farmers, foresters, fishermen	84	77
II	Miners and quarrymen	116	137
III	Gas, coke and chemicals makers	123	117
IV	Glass and ceramics makers	128	94
V	Furnace, forge, foundry, rolling mill workers	155	116
VI	Electrical and electronic workers	101	102
VII	Engineering and allied trades workers n.e.c.	118	111
VIII	Woodworkers	113	93
IX	Leather workers	104	88
X	Textile workers	88	102
XI	Clothing workers	104	91
XII	Food, drink and tobacco workers	129	104
XIII	Paper and printing workers	86	107
XIV	Makers of other products	96	112
XV	Construction workers	144	113
XVI	Painters and decorators	139	110
XVII	Drivers of stationary engines, cranes, etc.	113	125
XVIII	Labourers n.e.c.	146	133
XIX	Transport and communications workers	128	115
XX	Warehousemen, storekeepers, packers, bottlers	115	105
XXI	Clerical workers	79	87
XXII	Sales workers	85	91
XXIII	Service, sport and recreation workers	120	100
XXIV	Administrators and managers	60	76
XXV	Professional, technical workers, artists	51	66

* Observed proportion currently smoking cigarettes as percentage of expected proportion, standardised for age

TEXT-FIGURE 9.—Relationship between the average smoking habits in the 25 British occupational orders and the lung cancer mortality ratios of men at ages 15–64 in those occupations. (Fox, 1978; reprinted with permission of Her Majesty's Stationery Office and A. J. Fox.) *This correlation suggests that allowance for the effects of smoking is necessary before specific occupational lung cancer hazards can be assessed unbiasedly.*

tion of the available information can easily substitute different proportions and perhaps arrive at a more correct conclusion on the basis of freshly accumulated data.

First we have to decide how to classify cancers such as the lip and skin cancers produced by exposure to UV light associated with work in the open air, cancers of the upper respiratory and digestive tract due to the consumption of alcohol associated with work in bars, restaurants, and (in some circumstances) the manufacture of alcoholic drink, cancer of the cervix uteri in prostitutes due to intercourse with many men, and cancer of the breast in nuns due to the avoidance of pregnancy. As these are not the sort of cancers that are commonly termed "occupational," we should perhaps omit them, although we do so reluctantly. Secondly, we must decide what proportion of cancers to attribute to the occupational use of ionizing radiations. The experience accumulating from observation of the survivors of the atomic bomb explosions at Hiroshima and Nagasaki and of patients treated by radiotherapy strongly suggests that ionizing radiations can cause cancer in nearly all organs of the body and that some small effect is produced even by small doses and by doses given at low dose rates (*see* below for references). A figure based on the total incidence of cancer must, therefore, be added to the sum of the site-specific cancers due to occupational causes to allow for occupational exposure to these radiations.

Turning to other factors, we begin by classifying some types of cancer as never having been proved to be due to occupational causes at all. These are listed in table 17 with the numbers recorded nationally in 1977.

TABLE 17.—*Cancers that are not known to be produced by occupational hazards*[a]

Type of cancer	No. of deaths recorded in 1978 (United States)	
	Male	Female
Lip	130	28
Tongue	1,338	583
Pharynx	2,754	985
Small intestine	352	361
Gallbladder and bile ducts	1,612	2,877
Melanoma[b]	2,476	1,758
Breast	280	34,329
Cervix uteri	—	5,099
Other uterine cancers	—	5,773
Ovary	—	10,803
Other female genital organs[c]	—	1,095
Male genital organs other than prostate	806	—
Eye	164	158
Thyroid	351	672
Myeloma	3,123	2,978
Sub-total, above sites	13,386	67,499

[a] Excluding UV light and ionizing radiations (*see* text).
[b] Assumed to be 70% of all deaths due to skin cancer. Occupations involving regular outdoor work are associated with *lower* melanoma risks [Lee and Strickland (1980)].
[c] Malignant, benign, or unspecified.

TABLE 18.—*Cancers that possibly may be produced by occupational hazards*

Type of cancer	No. of deaths recorded in 1978 (United States)	
	Male	Female
Mouth	1,599	924
Esophagus	5,552	2,030
Stomach	8,529	5,923
Colon and rectum	25,696	27,573
Pancreas	11,010	9,767
Connective tissue	815	843
Kidney[a]	4,809	2,916
Brain[b]	6,737	5,996
Hodgkin's disease	1,249	916
Non-Hodgkin's lymphoma[c]	7,088	6,324
Sub-total, above sites	73,084	63,212
Postulated due to occupational hazards	731	316

[a] Includes ureter and urethra.
[b] Benign, unspecified, or malignant tumors of brain or other nerves.
[c] Excluding myeloma.

Another group of cancers may include a small proportion due to occupational exposure, but the evidence is weak or inconclusive. These types are listed in table 18, and in the absence of definite evidence we have allowed token proportions of 1% of male cases and 0.5% of female cases as due to occupational exposure. Finally, many types of cancer can certainly or almost certainly be produced by occupational hazards under defined conditions. These types are listed in table 19.

Attribution of particular proportions can be made with some confidence only in the case of cancer of the bladder, which has been the subject of several special studies because some occupations have engendered a very large risk of bladder cancer. These studies have provided estimates of the proportions of cases due to occupational exposure in men and women, respectively, of 18 and 6% (Cole et al., 1972), of 5 and 2% (Davies et al., 1976), and in the study most representative of the whole United States (Hoover et al., 1980), of 8% for both sexes combined. For bladder cancer, figures of 10% in men and 5% in women may seem large but are not likely to be far out.

A large percentage of cancers of the lung is also attributable to occupational factors, as several major occupations are known to involve or to have involved causes of the disease. Asbestos is the most outstanding example known, and the data discussed in appendix F suggest that it may cause some 5% of all present-day lung cancers. Occupational exposure to the combustion products of fossil fuels is also common (*see* table 16), and even though the relative risks involved are seldom high, the numbers of workers exposed are so large that it may be responsible for another 5% of all male cases. It cannot, however, have been responsible for many cases in women, as the exposed jobs have been heavy and dirty (e.g., in coal gasification or steel foundries), and few women have been employed to do

TABLE 19.—*Cancers that definitely can be produced by occupational hazards*

Type of cancer	No. of deaths recorded in 1978		Cancer deaths ascribed to occupational hazards in 1978 (United States)			
			Male		Female	
	Male	Female	No. ascribed	% ascribed	No. ascribed	% ascribed
Mesentery and peritoneum[a]	652	697	98	15	35	5
Liver[b] and intrahepatic bile ducts	1,812	984	72	4	10	1
Larynx	2,909	550	58	2	6	1
Lung[b,c]	71,006	24,080	10,651	15	1,204	5
Pleura, nasal sinuses, and remaining respiratory sites	857	496	214	25	25	5
Bone[b]	997	740	40	4	7	1
Skin other than melanoma	1,061	753	106	10	15	2
Prostate	21,674	—	217	1	—	—
Bladder	6,771	3,078	677	10	154	5
Leukemia	8,683	6,708	868	10	335	5
Other and unspecified[d] cancers	15,445	14,821	1,045	6.8	185	1.2
Sub-total,[e] above sites	131,867	52,907	14,046	—	1,976	—

[a] Includes peritoneal mesotheliomas, but also cancer of "unspecified digestive sites."

[b] Includes many misdiagnosed secondary cancers from other sites.

[c] Assumed to include some miscertified cases of pleural mesothelioma.

[d] Chiefly unspecified, so the percentages have been chosen to match the percentages ($\male$, 13,732/202,892; $\female$, 2,107/168,797) in the aggregate of all specified sites in tables 17–19 that we have attributed to occupational factors. (Includes all remaining tumors of malignant, benign, or unspecified histology.)

[e] Our estimate of the total effects of occupational factors is the sum of the subtotals in tables 17–19, i.e., 14,777/218,337 $\male$ and 2,292/183,618 $\female$.

them. Other recognized hazards have affected only small groups and we have, therefore, attributed to occupational factors total proportions of 15% of male and 5% of female cases of lung cancer.

This proportion for male cases is intermediate between the figures estimated for Los Angeles County by Pike et al. (1979; *see also* Menck and Henderson, 1976) and those obtained by Hammond and Garfinkel (1980) for the million Americans in the ACS prospective study. The former authors estimated that the proportion of lung cancers attributable to blue-collar occupations might be as high as 36%, but they gave this figure tentatively, qualifying it with the statement that the occupational differences "are likely to be partly due to unmeasured differences in patterns of cigarette use such as tar content, inhalation, and butt length." We have discounted it altogether, partly because differences in smoking habits were allowed for by subdivision into only three broad groups, but mainly because the information about individuals was obtained in different and potentially non-comparable ways (from the spouses, children, and siblings of the cases, but from the controls themselves). The ACS data lead to a much lower estimate based on the assumption that major occupational hazards have occurred only in the presence of recognizable fumes, mists, or dust. After standardization for smoking, the mortality from lung cancer was only 14% greater in men who gave a history of such exposure at work (including exposure to asbestos) than in men who did not. Since only 38% of lung cancer deaths occurred in men who gave a positive history, the total contribution of these factors to the production of the disease appears to have been 4.6%.

An estimate derived in this way may be too low for three reasons: the diluting effect of random errors, the possibility that the ACS population was biased against the inclusion of blue-collar workers, and the possibility that some undiscovered carcinogenic effects may exist in industries in which there are no recognized dusts, mists, or fumes. We have, therefore, adhered to the proportions previously suggested, but we suspect that they are a little high.

Several of the remaining types of cancer listed in table 19 are likely to include only a small proportion of occupational cases, as the hazards are either small or affect only a minute proportion of the total population (e.g., cancer of the prostate in cadmium workers, cancer of the bone in luminizers, and cancer of the larynx in mustard gas manufacturers and perhaps in nickel refiners). No firm evidence exists on which exact estimates can be made, and we have allocated proportions of between 1 and 10% of cases of the remaining types of cancer on the crude and unreliable basis of our interpretation of the literature and clinical impression.

Finally, we have added 58 deaths as a result of occupational exposure to ionizing radiations on the same basis as that recently adopted by Jablon and Bailar (1980): that is, on the assumption that the effect of ionizing radiations is proportional to the dose received, that the life-time risk of fatal cancer per rem whole-body dose is about 250 per million people, and that the total dose received by all men and women occupationally exposed to ionizing radiations is about 233,000 rems/year. In making these assumptions we have accepted the estimate of the effect of ionizing radiations that was made by the United Nations

Scientific Committee on the Effects of Atomic Radiation (UNSCEAR) (1977) and the estimate of the number of persons occupationally exposed and the doses they received that was made by the Interagency Task Force on the Health Effects of Ionizing Radiation (1979) under the chairmanship of Dr. Libassi. The UNSCEAR estimate of the number of cancers produced per rem is within the range of the effects estimated by the Advisory Committee on the Biological Effect of Ionizing Radiations (1979) of the National Academy of Sciences and the National Research Council (that is, 70–353 fatalities/million/rem) and is very close to the independent estimate of one of us (R. D.) who has conducted research into the effects of ionizing radiations on humans since 1955. The much larger effects recently suggested by some investigators do not stand up to critical examination and derive chiefly from an analysis by inappropriate statistical methods of the data on the workers at the Hanford Nuclear plant. When these data are analyzed according to standard efficient epidemiological methods (Darby and Reissland, 1981), there is nothing in them to suggest that the estimates of total cancer risk made by the committees referred to above need to be revised. The only unusual feature was that the excess risk was chiefly of myelomatosis, possibly because some particular source(s) or type(s) of radiation may have a specific effect on the risk of myelomatosis (*see* Cuzick, 1981). This suggestion should, however, be regarded as no more than a hypothesis that requires testing by further inquiry.

The proportion of cancer deaths that we have tentatively attributed to occupational causes is, therefore, about 17,000 out of 400,000, i.e., about 4% of all U.S. cancer deaths. In developing this argument we have given precise numbers not because we believe that they are individually accurate—though we believe that the final conclusion is unlikely to be out in either direction by more than a factor of about two—but so that our numbers may be corrected as further information is obtained from reasonably representative studies of individual types of cancer, like the information which has recently been obtained for cancer of the bladder. Since by far the largest contribution to our estimate is 11,000-odd lung cancers, the chief need is for a nationally representative case–control study of lung cancer in relation to smoking and occupation.[35] Such a study might reveal unsuspected occupational hazards, and until it is done something like twofold uncertainty about the true magnitude of the occupa-

tional cancer problem is likely to persist. However, since in the late 1970's some hundreds of mesotheliomas a year were due to asbestos, at least a few thousand other cancers must have been attributable to asbestos (*see* appendix F), so asbestos must account for 1 or 2% of all cancer deaths. Although different figures may, of course, apply to other countries, the minimum proportion of all current U.S. cancer deaths attributable to occupation can hardly be less than 2 or 3%. This proportion is small, but cancer is so common and the U.S. population so large that even 2% of cancer deaths amounts to more than 8,000 deaths in the United States every year. Occupational cancer, moreover, tends to be concentrated among relatively small groups of people among whom the risk of developing the disease may be quite large, and such risks can usually be reduced, or even eliminated, once they have been identified. The detection of occupational hazards should therefore have a higher priority in any program of cancer prevention than their proportional importance might suggest.

5.7 Pollution

The air that we breathe, the water we drink, the food we eat, and the earth on which we live are all polluted to some extent with the products of human activity, and we shall discuss the first three of these problems separately. Air pollution has, in certain circumstances, been so intense that it reduced visibility in towns to a few yards and caused the deaths of some thousands of Londoners in December 1952, and a substantial epidemic of poisoning was caused in Japan by the industrial discharge of mercury into the sea (where it was ingested by shellfish that were subsequently eaten). Such gross pollution is now largely, if not entirely, eliminated from the American environment, except in the immediate vicinity of old chemical waste dumps, but we are left with lesser degrees of pollution that may, perhaps, produce ill effects, especially if human exposure is prolonged throughout a large part of the life-span.

The effects of low levels of pollutants on the incidence of chronic diseases such as cancer are peculiarly difficult to observe directly since many different pollutants are likely to be present in each geographic area, the absolute risks from each are likely to be low (and not evident for some decades), and although different areas are exposed to different pollutants there may be little variation in the degrees of exposure of different individuals within particular areas. Consequently, one generally has to rely on two indirect sources of data. First, have high levels of chronic exposure to a particular pollutant or group of pollutants (usually in an industrial context) ever been studied? If so, we may be able to extrapolate downward from the known risks of high chronic exposure (or, in the case where high chronic exposure produced no apparent effect, to extrapolate downward from the known upper limit to its risks) to say something useful about the approximate effects of chronic exposure

---

[35] One of us performed such a study on 1,465 matched pairs with a special emphasis on occupational causes in five English cities more than 30 years ago. The recognized hazard of work in coal-gas retort houses was confirmed, but no new occupational hazards were discovered. Such studies are generally not difficult to conduct as long as bias is not introduced into the data by asking leading questions (Doll and Hill, 1952; Doll, 1953), or into the analysis by failing to standardize for smoking, etc., or by placing undue (*see* text) trust in data-derived hypotheses.

levels 100 or 1,000 times lower.[36] Second, are particular pollutants, mutagenic or otherwise, active in any short-term laboratory tests or in long-term animal cancer tests, and, if so, how potent do they seem to be? As discussed in section 4.2, although it is not at present justifiable to jump from any such potency estimates to a quantitative assessment of human risk, they may nevertheless help reduce the list of pollutants to worry about from a few thousand to a few dozen. Indeed, the chief difficulty in discussing the whole area of pollution is that the variety of possible routes and forms of pollution is so enormous that no one can pretend to have serious expertise about all of them. In this section more than any other we must therefore touch on areas in which others have studied the available evidence more carefully than we ever have (at which points we have tried to draw attention to National Academy of Science or other reviews) and on areas which are so much at the margins of scientific knowledge that no one is reliably informed. In both circumstances the general perspectives discussed in section 4 (on the lack of general epidemic increases in U.S. non-respiratory cancer rates and on the use of laboratory tests for priority setting rather than for risk assessment) may help to achieve a reasonable balance between complacency and hysteria, neither of which seems to be currently indicated.

Air Pollution

Many of the agents listed in table 16 escape into the ambient atmosphere in the course of industrial activity and constitute a potential source of carcinogenicity. Those that escape in largest amounts are polycyclic hydrocarbons (formed by the combustion of fossil fuel and the refining of petroleum), arsenic, asbestos, and radioactive elements. That these (or other) substances in urban air might be responsible for some cases of lung cancer was first suggested when it was realized that the mortality from lung cancer was almost invariably greater in large towns than in the countryside. It is clear, however, that these substances acting by themselves can be responsible for only a small proportion of all cases of the disease, since the mortality rate among non-smokers is extremely low, irrespective of the area in which they live (reviewed by Doll, 1978). It is possible however (though by no means certain) that some pollutant(s) of urban air may interact with cigarette smoke to increase the incidence of cancer over

and above that which would be expected by the action of tobacco alone, as was noted in section 4.4.

Some investigators have attempted to estimate the effect of pollutants by comparing the lung cancer mortality rates in different areas and "making allowance" for differences in smoking habits by retrospective inquiry of the amount smoked by representative residents. We doubt, however, whether it is possible in this way to disentangle the effects of smoking and environmental pollution, especially in those studies that have examined cancer rates only within categories of men with such broadly similar smoking habits as non-smokers (including ex-smokers), current smokers smoking 20 cigarettes a day or less, and current smokers smoking more. Such broad classes are hardly likely to take account of differences in a habit which may affect the incidence of lung cancer by up to fortyfold sufficiently accurately for a twofold urban–rural difference to be estimated with certainty.

Effects of Past Cigarette Use on Current Urban–Rural Lung Cancer Differences

The reasons for uncertainty deserve some detailed discussion, for if they are overlooked a misleading impression of the hazards of air pollution may be engendered. The key observation is that lung cancer risks among cigarette smokers in middle and old age depend very strongly on the exact age at which cigarette smoking began. For example, delay of the onset of cigarette smoking in the late teens or early twenties by just a couple of years may reduce the risk of lung cancer at age 60 or 70 by as much as 20% (*see* text-fig. E1 on page 1292). Therefore, lung cancer risks in cities and in rural areas depend strongly not only on what old people now smoke, but also on what they smoked in early adult life half a century or so ago. If cigarette smoking by *young* adults was somewhat more prevalent (in terms of percentages of serious cigarette smokers or numbers of cigarettes per smoker) in cities than in rural areas during the first half of this century, this alone would engender a substantial excess of lung cancer today when cigarette-smoking city dwellers are compared with cigarette-smoking country dwellers. The smoking of substantial numbers of cigarettes was an extremely uncommon habit in all countries in about 1900, while by 1950 it had become common throughout the developed world.

While any new habit is in the process of becoming adopted by society (e.g., the use of various drugs today), it is likely that its prevalence among young adults will be greater in cities than in rural areas.[37] In

---

[36] This procedure is obviously very uncertain, but it seems reasonable to expect that for most carcinogens a reduction of the dose rate by 1,000 should reduce the attributable risks by a factor of about 1,000 in many cases and by a factor of more than 1,000 in many others, often without any absolute threshold of risk and without materially increasing the average age at which any attributable cancers will arise (Guess et al., 1977). However, it is difficult to make due allowance for the difference in effect between perhaps 20 years of industrial exposure and perhaps 70 years of environmental exposure, and the latter might be as much as one or two orders of magnitude more dangerous per unit of daily dose.

[37] In confirmation of this, a survey conducted by *Fortune* magazine in 1935 found the respective percentages of men and women who smoked any form of tobacco to be 61 and 31% in large cities, as against 44 and 9% in rural areas. Since many rural men smoked only pipes and/or cigars (which have relatively much less effect on lung cancer than cigarettes), the urban–rural differences between the percentages who smoked *cigarettes* between World Wars I and II were probably very marked among the young of both sexes.

appendix E we discuss in detail the effects of differences in cigarette usage in early adult life on the lung cancer risks many decades later among men who would all, in later life, describe themselves as "long-term regular cigarette smokers of one pack of cigarettes per day." Because of such effects, one must anticipate, even if air pollution were completely irrelevant to the carcinogenicity of cigarettes, to find that urban smokers now have greater lung cancer risks than do apparently similar rural smokers, at least in studies of populations who still live in the type of area (urban or rural) where they grew up. This should, of course, also hold in countries other than the United States, and it is noteworthy that urban–rural differences in countries such as Finland and Norway where the cities have not been heavily polluted are of a similar size to the urban–rural differences in Britain and the United States. Given these likely sources of substantial bias, however, it is remarkable how small urban–rural differences in lung cancer are among current smokers with similar *current* habits. For example, Hammond and Garfinkel (1980) report a prospective study in which, among men who in 1959 reported having lived in the same neighborhood for at least 10 years, 1,510 died of lung cancer between 1959 and 1972. From these data three roughly equal groups can be compared: a) city dwellers in metropolitan areas (likely to be most heavily exposed), b) people living in rural parts of non-metropolitan areas (likely to be least heavily exposed), and c) all others, standardizing for age and for six categories of *current* smoking. If the risk ratio of a is made to be 100%, the risk ratios of the others are 85% for b and 94% for c. These differences do not allow for differences attributable to occupational hazards but even so are not large, and much or all of them might be due to the expected effects of early cigarette usage. The authors allowed for occupation by examining separately men exposed and not exposed to dust, fumes, etc. and concluded that their data offer "little or no support to the hypothesis that urban air pollution has an important effect on lung cancer."[38]

In Britain, we have monitored the smoking habits and mortality of male doctors (Doll and Peto, 1976) and can relate their place of residence (as adults) in 1951 to their subsequent lung cancer mortality. No relationship whatsoever was observed,[39] but it should

be noted that all were educated in big cities and may have lived as children in areas different from those they inhabited in 1951.

All such comparisons, especially in the United States, are rendered difficult because people move about so much. Since emigration is a much less common activity than moving house, this difficulty may be reduced by comparing different countries which differ markedly in air pollution but in which the men have smoked cigarettes for a very long time. The obvious comparison for this purpose is between Britain, which was on average more polluted than the United States, and Finland, which has never been heavily polluted. Between the two World Wars, the average sales of manufactured cigarettes per adult were similar in Finland and in Britain (and so cigarette usage per young man may also have been similar), and British and Finnish lung cancer mortality among people who had been young men between the two wars has been almost identical in recent years (and has exceeded U.S. rates; *see* appendix E).

This international comparison is crude in that past and present exposure of Finnish and English lungs to cigarette smoke is not exactly known, but it is reassuring in that purely statistical errors are negligible and that the populations being compared have been exposed *throughout life* to very different mean levels of air pollution without apparent effect.

Direct epidemiological comparison of countries or of urban and rural residents thus shows, as long as the unavoidable biases are borne in mind when commenting on the results, little or no effect of air pollution. To distinguish between "little" and "no" from such direct comparisons is not of course possible, as any real effects will probably be undetectably small, while even if there are no real effects it is impossible to prove a negative.

Extrapolation From Known Effects of Heavy Exposure

An indirect method is to extrapolate from occupational studies in which the mortality from lung cancer has been found to be abnormally high, and measurements have been made of the concentration of certain carcinogens in the respired air. This method was used by Pike et al. (1975) to estimate the effect of urban pollution with polycyclic hydrocarbons from the experience of men who made coal gas in Britain (and similar deductions can be made from the experience of roofers working with pitch and asphalt in the United States: Hammond et al., 1976). Pike and his colleagues concluded that the pollution characterized by 1 ng benzo[a]pyrene/m^3 of city air might result in the annual production of 4 cases/million men 40–74 years of age with average British smoking habits. This calculation does not assume that benzo[a]pyrene is the only relevant carcinogen, but rather that the important carcinogenic agents in air polluted by the combustion products of fuel are qualitatively similar in the retort houses of gasworks and in city streets and that the

---

[38] It is uncertain whether these differences would be much reduced by inquiring about early cigarette usage and standardizing for the replies, as they would be subject to such large random errors as indicators of actual exposure of the lungs to smoke in early adult life as to prevent complete elimination of the confounding effects of interest (*see* appendix B.14: Two properties of multiple regression analysis *in* Fletcher et al., 1976).

[39] Unpublished data. After standardizing for smoking and age, we would have *expected* 153.65, 88.04, 109.46, and 78.85 deaths in conurbations, large towns (50,000–100,000), small towns (<50,000), and rural areas, respectively. We *observed* 152, 94, 108, and 76 lung cancer deaths (respective ratios: 0.99, 1.07, 0.99, and 0.96).

quantity of carcinogenic agents varies, in both situations, in approximate proportion to the amount of benzo[a]pyrene. As much as 30 or 40 ng of benzo[a]pyrene/m³ was commonly present in the air of big cities, and the estimate of Pike et al. would lead to the conclusion that atmospheric pollution, in conjunction with cigarette smoke, might have contributed to some 10% of all cases of lung cancer in big cities (and so a few percent of lung cancer in the country as a whole, i.e., about 1% of all cancer). A symposium at the Karolinska Institute in Stockholm in 1977 reached a less precise conclusion that, however, indicated an effect of much the same size: that is, that "Combustion products of fossil fuels in ambient air, probably acting together with cigarette smoke, have been responsible for cases of lung cancer in large urban areas, the numbers produced being of the order of 5–10 cases per 100,000 males per year" (Cederlöf et al., 1978), which would again account for about 10% of lung cancer in big cities or 1% of all cancer. These crude estimates probably provide the best basis for the formation of policy. It should be noted, however, that the concentration of benzo[a]pyrene in town air in Britain and the United States is now commonly an order of magnitude less than it used to be (Lawther and Waller, 1978) and that on this basis the recent contribution of atmospheric benzo[a]pyrene and associated combustion products (including both gas-phase and particulate matter) to the production of lung cancer is unlikely to account for more than 1% of cases of cancer of the lung in the future, and so will then account for only a fraction of 1% of all cancer.

Air Pollutants Other Than Combustion Products

Similar calculations for arsenic (Albert, 1978) and asbestos (Doll, 1977) suggest that the current and future contribution from atmospheric pollution by these agents should be minute, although there may be exceptions where the atmosphere around a particular factory is abnormally contaminated (Blot and Fraumeni, 1975). For asbestos, it appears that sufficient amounts can be carried home on the clothes of asbestos workers to create a hazard of mesothelioma for household contacts, 37 of whom have been reported to develop this normally very rare disease (Anderson et al., 1976). The amount commonly present in town air is, however, three or four orders of magnitude less than the most stringent regulations currently permit at work, and the risk to the general public from this source is unlikely to increase appreciably the total number of cancers attributable to other forms of air pollution.

Under the heading of atmospheric pollution, we may also include the effect on the general population of the mining and milling of uranium and other radioactive ores, the pollution caused by the nuclear energy industry (although not all of it is atmospheric), and the radioactive fallout due to past testing of nuclear weapons. On the assumptions that we made in relation to occupational hazards (section 5.6), we estimate this to be the production of about 590 fatal cancers/year.

No other air pollutants seem likely to produce more cancer than arsenic, asbestos, and radioactivity, except perhaps for the chlorofluorocarbons that have been used extensively as refrigerants and aerosol propellants. These persist in the atmosphere and, it is thought, will eventually reach the stratosphere where they will react with ozone, reduce its concentration, and hence permit more UV light to reach the surface of the earth. If this happens, the incidence of skin cancer, including the relatively fatal melanoma of the skin, must be expected to rise. The arguments, which are complex and based on a number of unproved assumptions about physical and chemical processes, have been reviewed by a panel of the National Research Council (1976), and we are not in a position to comment on their conclusion. We would note only that oxides of nitrogen released as a result of the cultivation of the soil and the extensive use of nitrate fertilizers may have a similar but smaller effect (National Research Council, 1978) or an opposite one (Turco et al., 1978) and that much more research is needed before the sum of the effects of all pollutants on the ozone layer can be predicted with confidence. An increase of up to 20% in the mortality from skin cancer might be produced by these agents in the future (0.3% of all cancer deaths), but the present contribution is likely to be at least one order of magnitude less.

Drinking Water

The situation with regard to pollution of drinking water is rather more obscure. Analytical techniques now permit the detection of chemicals at concentrations well below 1 ppb (and further rapid improvements in sensitivity must be anticipated), and consequently, many chemicals have been found to contaminate drinking water supplies. Some of these may be classed on the basis of laboratory tests as carcinogens or mutagens (or suspected carcinogens or mutagens), and the possibility that they may constitute a material hazard to health has been examined by the National Academy of Sciences (1977). As a result of its report, the EPA has promulgated a regulation establishing a "maximum contaminant level" of 100 μg total trihalomethanes/liter for all community water systems serving 10,000 persons or more and adding a disinfectant in the treatment of their water supplies.

The EPA did not claim that drinking water, as now supplied in the United States, had been proved to cause cancer. However, human exposure to water pollutants may be prolonged over so many decades that even weak carcinogenic stimuli might in principle have material effects, and the evidence that they might do so includes:

a) There is activity in short-term carcinogenicity tests or animal cancer tests of certain pollutants (or, equivalently, there is an excess of tumors in marine animals that live in polluted waters).

b) Some pollutants are present that are known or believed to cause cancer in humans if large amounts are ingested (e.g., asbestos from industrial activity, from asbestos cement water pipes, or from the passage of groundwater through natural asbestos-rich rock formations; radionuclides from industrial activity or natural sources; arsenic; and vinyl chloride from PVC water pipes).

There are human population studies that report positive correlations between the amounts of certain contaminants and mortality from certain cancers (for review, see Crump and Guess, 1980).

We have already discussed earlier in this section and in section 4.2 possible ways in which laboratory data may be used for priority setting (if not for quantitative risk estimation), and we shall therefore pass over *a*. Under *b*, with the possible exception of asbestos in a few water supplies, we know of no established human carcinogen that is ever present in sufficient quantities in large U.S. public water supplies to account for any material percentage of the total risk of cancer. The observations on U.S. asbestos workers reported by Selikoff et al. (1979) suggest that occupational exposure to asbestos dust leads to an increased risk of cancer of the gastrointestinal tract, presumably through ingestion of mucus containing most of the asbestos dust from the respiratory passages. If, due to some local industrial or natural geological circumstances, the numbers of asbestos fibers per liter are within a few orders of magnitude of the daily numbers ingested by Selikoff's workers (and especially if these numbers include some with comparable physical characteristics), then the likely benefits from filtering them out or otherwise avoiding them may be estimated reasonably sensibly by assuming approximate proportionality of risk to dose rate, despite the disparity in the number of decades of exposure at work and to water. However, it is again not plausible that any material percentage of the total number of cancers in the whole United States derives from this source.

Turning finally to *c* (epidemiology), the interpretation of the correlation[40] studies is at present open to question. Similar studies have been carried out over the years in many other fields (for example, showing that "contamination" of drinking water by calcium appears to decrease the risk of heart disease: Crawford et al., 1968) but have rarely been regarded as constituting anything more than hypotheses to be tested by more specific work, because of the difficulty of obtaining truly relevant data (relating to long-past exposure of the actual individuals concerned) and of eliminating the effects of concomitant variation. (The specific difficulties inherent in correlation studies of cancer and

drinking water composition have been emphasized by Hogan et al., 1979.) Analyses that took account of other important variables and were consistent from one region to another in pointing to specific effects on one or other specific type of cancer would carry some weight, but most of the analyses have not met these criteria.

Suggestive Evidence of Possible Effects of Chlorination

The chief exceptions are the studies by Cantor et al. (1978) and various others suggesting a relationship between the concentrations of halogenated organic matter in water and mortality from cancers of the bladder and, possibly, the large intestine. When water is chlorinated to kill germs, much of the plant debris and other organic matter naturally present in it is also halogenated, resulting in a complex mixture of halogenated compounds at levels of up to some parts per million (depending principally on the concentration of organic matter that was originally present). Many specific halogenated compounds have been found to cause tumors in laboratory animals and some have also done so in man. It is therefore reasonable to inquire whether lifelong exposure to the non-specific mixture present in water that has been chlorinated has any material effect on the risks from any type of tumor. If the large NCI case–control study of bladder cancer that is currently being analyzed indicates any substantial relationship among individuals with the concentration of such compounds in drinking water (or if any really well-controlled[41] studies of cancer of the large intestine do so), then this will lend urgency to similar studies of many other types of tumor. However, in view of our previous estimate of some thousands of cancers which urban air pollution may cause by enhancing the carcinogenicity of cigarettes, it seems on present evidence that any effects of drinking water pollution will probably be *relatively* less important. If this is so, then they will not materially affect the total percentage of cancer deaths to be attributed to "pollution." But it has to be borne in mind that the long duration of exposure to any traces of carcinogens that drinking water may contain will enhance any effects they might have.

Lack of Evidence for Effects of Fluoridation

We have not, it will be noted, paid any attention in this assessment to the claim that fluoridation of water increases the risk of cancer. The evidence that has been

---

[40] By "correlation" studies we mean studies in which estimated cancer mortality rates in particular populations are correlated with the estimated composition of the drinking water in those entire populations. Misleadingly extreme significance levels (e.g., Kanarek et al., 1980) may arise in such studies if all sources of variation other than Poisson variation in the number of cases of cancer are ignored, but these will be moderated or eliminated if proper account is taken of the variation in estimated cancer onset rates between communities and of the likely similarities between neighboring communities in both cancer rates and water composition.

---

[41] In view of the relevance of environmental and life-style factors to many diseases other than cancer (and especially the possibility that contamination of drinking water by magnesium or, as Crawford et al., 1968, suggest, calcium may protect against vascular disease), the use of deaths from non-neoplastic causes as "controls" in case-control studies of cancer (Alavanja et al., 1978) may lead to uncertainties of interpretation of any apparent positive, null, or inverse associations.

advanced for this claim has been examined in detail by the National Cancer Institute, the Royal Statistical Society in Britain, and one of us (R. D.) as well as by many other individual scientists and has no scientific basis whatsoever. The appearance of an above-average increase in the crude death rates from cancer that has been observed in some U.S. cities following fluoridation is entirely accounted for by the demographic changes in the sex, age, and ethnic composition of the populations of the cities. In New Zealand, fluoridation happens to have been followed by a relative decrease in age-standardized cancer mortality (Goodall et al., 1980), but nobody seems to have claimed that fluoridation prevents cancer.

Pollution of Food

Contamination of food by bacterial, fungal, and other natural products has been dealt with under "Diet" (section 5.3). Food can also be contaminated by a wide variety of industrial products ranging from heavy metals through pesticide residues to substances that leach out of packaging and the combustion products of fossil fuels that precipitate from the atmosphere, while fish that will be eaten can be contaminated by various types of marine pollution including industrial effluents, precipitates from the atmosphere, and spills of oil.

Polycyclic hydrocarbons are found widely in all sorts of food, sometimes even in the same amounts as in charcoal-broiled meats and smoked ham (i.e., up to 15 μg benzo[a]pyrene/kg net weight) (GESAMP, 1977; Dunn and Fee, 1979; King, 1977). The extreme amounts that have occasionally been reported in shellfish and finfish from relatively polluted waters (up to 1,000 μg benzo[a]pyrene/kg) might be a cause for concern if they constituted a regular item of diet. It is, however, difficult to produce cancer experimentally by feeding animals polycyclic hydrocarbons by mouth, and the cancers that can be produced (in the forestomach of the mouse and, with very large doses of DMBA, in the breast) either affect organs that are not represented in humans or seem to be produced by mechanisms that would not be brought into play by much smaller doses (such as disturbances of immune or hormonal status). More importantly, men who made coal gas or worked as roofers (*see* section 5.6) and swallowed large amounts of tar with their respiratory mucus did not develop any excess of gastrointestinal cancer.

The average amount of vinyl chloride absorbed by the general population via food wrapped in PVC is several million times less per day than that inspired by the early manufacturers of PVC (Barnes, 1976; MAFF, 1978) and so will have produced few or no cases of angiosarcoma of the liver in the entire United States.

Some pesticides are long lasting, are (or were) found in food, and have accumulated in substantial amounts in human fat[42] (e.g., DDT and dieldrin). It is notable, however, that there has been no general increase in the incidence of liver tumors in developed countries since the long-lasting pesticides were introduced, despite the fact that hepatomas are the principal type of cancer to have been reported in laboratory animals under experimental conditions. (Data on U.S. trends in liver cancer mortality are discussed in appendix D. At ages under 65, at which death certification is most reliable, there was during 1968–78 a non-significant increase in female mortality and a non-significant decrease in male mortality, although liver cancer remains virtually incurable.) According to the International Agency for Research on Cancer Working Group (1980), the evidence of animal carcinogenesis of those that have been reviewed is at most "limited," and the extent to which they should be regarded as potential human carcinogens is uncertain. Some pesticides which leave residues in the form of secondary amines could perhaps constitute a hazard if the formation of nitrosamine in the stomach proves to be a cause of cancer, as discussed in section 5.3. Others, according to recent Swedish reports (*see* Hardell et al., 1981), might be responsible for some lymphomas and sarcomas.

For our present limited purpose (of estimating the proportion of *current* cancer mortality avoidable in various ways), the occurrence of pesticides as dietary pollutants seems unimportant. However, this does not imply that no modification of current practices is advisable. Obviously, where human exposure can be avoided without undue cost, perhaps by different or more limited pesticide practices or by the use of some alternative methods of control, it would seem prudent to do so. [The recent NAS report (CPEAP, 1980) on the Environmental Protection Agency's pesticide regulation program provides a thoughtful and balanced account of how, with the limited information that will in practice be available, pesticide regulation might be approached.]

Total Effects of Air, Water, and Food Pollution

We have tried in this review to take account of the main industrial pollutants of air, water, and food of which we have any personal knowledge. Many others must exist, and it is not impossible that they interact with one another even though present in only minute amounts, some perhaps acting as promoters rather than initiators. We prefer, however, not to speculate about their harmful effects in the absence of evidence and have therefore limited our estimate of the cancer

---

[42] Certain substances are stored much more readily in the adipose tissue of "yellow-fat" animals such as man than of "white-fat" animals such as laboratory rodents. Whether, for substances that are hazardous to both mice and men, the more comparable index of exposure is generally the amount ingested per kilogram of body weight or the amount stored per gram of fat is unclear; if the former, then human exposure to some substances may be relatively lower than comparison of adipose tissue concentrations in mouse and man would suggest. However, there is no guarantee that this will be so.

hazards from pollution to a token figure of 2%, accounted for chiefly by the uncertain effect of the combustion products of fossil fuels in urban air. An upper limit is difficult to select until the role, if any, of halogenated compounds in drinking water is clarified, and the upper limit of 5% which we shall suggest in table 20 (on page 1256) is therefore rather arbitrary.

5.8 Industrial Products

Industrial products (excluding asbestos-containing products which we deal with elsewhere) such as detergents and other surfactants, hair dyes and other cosmetics, solid or foam plastics, paints, dyes, polishes, solvents, fabrics, and even the processed paper and the printer's ink in the present volume are a class of agents which are so numerous that we can only echo the uncertainty with which we discussed many pollutants in the previous section. It is possible that some such products are already causing, unnoticed, a number of today's cancers, and it is quite possible that, after prolonged exposure to them, some substantial risks will be detected in the future. For example, in mouse skin carcinogenesis surfactants (e.g., Tween 60) are potent promoting agents; permanent hair dyes currently contain as essential components substances such as 2,4-diaminoanisole which can damage DNA, and some of these components are also carcinogenic to laboratory rodents, as are many of the monomers of which plastics are made and by which the finished products are inevitably slightly contaminated; many of the halogenated solvents in common domestic, office, or industrial use (e.g., as degreasers) can cause mouse liver tumors, and so on. In general, for each product there is inadequate laboratory evidence and inadequate human evidence to know whether it is a health hazard or whether it is harmless. Rather than provide an inconclusive (and therefore tedious) review of each of several dozen products, we shall instead discuss what general sort of evidence it would be reasonable to seek.

First, as many different defined occupational groups as possible might routinely be monitored, for it often happens that if a product (e.g., asbestos) is significantly but undetectably hazardous to the general population, it will be detectably hazardous to those who manufacture it or work with it or with related agents.

Second, a large sample of young adults who develop various cancers might routinely be interviewed, along with suitable control subjects, in a permanent ongoing study into which the general scientific community could feed suggestions for possible questions to check, and which might be built into the ongoing SEER program. The reasons for including large numbers of cases of lung cancer in such a study have already been reviewed (comparison of effects of different types of cigarettes, estimation of lung cancer rate and effects of passive smoking among non-smokers, identification of new occupational hazards, and direct estimation of the much-disputed percentage of cancers due to occupa-

tional factors), and because of their theoretical importance or their close linkage with certain occupational factors, primary tumors of the bladder, liver, nasal sinuses, peritoneum, pleura, and scrotum should probably also be included.

Third, as discussed at some length in section 4.2, a very large number of substances could be subjected to various short-term tests to see which stand out clearly. (This may be a useful mechanism for reducing the number of substances to worry about from 10,000 to 100 and is already under way at the National Institute of Environmental Health Sciences under Dr. J. Drake.)

Fourth, when particular hypotheses are generated (for example, that hair dye may be carcinogenic), careful epidemiologic studies should be undertaken, especially if people can be found who have been exposed to the substance *regularly* for *many* years. There is at present such a gross lack of reliable human data on the relevance to humans of positive findings in short-term tests or animal feeding studies that even negative findings in careful, unbiased human studies are of considerable scientific interest. (Of course, any positive findings that may emerge are of even more interest.) However, there is a need for considerable care if such studies are to seek evidence concerning moderate risks, for the biases that are particularly inherent in poorly controlled epidemiology may considerably exceed the magnitude of the effects which one could plausibly hope to observe. This may be the case with hair dye use. Various components of "permanent" hair dyes are mutagenic in "Ames test" bacteria and can cause cancer when fed to laboratory animals. However, few people drink hair dyes, and if used in the normal way, only a fraction of 1% of the applied dose is absorbed systemically, which suggests that if there are any human risks from a few decades of normal use, they are likely to be small. The large epidemiological studies in which bias is least likely to obtrude have in our opinion not provided evidence of any material cancer risk arising, at least during the first 20 years of hair dye use (Kinlen et al., 1977; Hennekens et al., 1979). If no excess risk is observable even with more prolonged use, then this will give a somewhat reassuring perspective on any substantially smaller exposures to agents with comparable laboratory activity, while if any clearly measurable hazard does materialize, this will be a useful step toward a better perspective on such agents and might, of course, help people avoid that particular hazard.

Current trends in cancer incidence give no urgent cause for alarm, but many industrial products have been introduced so recently (and on such a large scale: *see* text-fig. 8 on page 1239) that even if they do prove hazardous or if they replace a previous hazard with a less hazardous product, their effects would not yet be apparent. Although we can attribute only a nominal "less than 1%" of all current cancer deaths to such products, we must reiterate our conclusion from some previous sections: There is too much ignorance for complacency to be justified.

5.9 Medicines and Medical Procedures

Among the few dozen agents and conditions listed as established human carcinogens in table 6 on page 1203, about a third have been used in the course of medical practice (cyclophosphamide, melphalan, arsenic, busulfan, chlornaphazine, immunosuppressive drugs, ionizing radiations, estrogens, phenacetin, polycyclic hydrocarbons, oxymetholone, steroid contraceptives, and UV light), and most of these 13 have been shown to cause cancer in humans only when used in this way (that is, all but arsenic, ionizing radiations, polycyclic hydrocarbons, and UV light). That so many carcinogenic agents should have been prescribed medically is not surprising when it is borne in mind that treatment often requires some modification of the metabolism of human cells and that sometimes it is intended to interfere with the DNA itself. (For this reason, it may well be that many more of the cytotoxic agents that have been or will be introduced to treat cancer are themselves carcinogens: *see* review by Harris, 1979). However, the possible production of cancer, although always an undesirable side effect, is not necessarily a bar to the use of a drug if the risk of loss of life due to the possible development of iatrogenic cancer is materially less than the chance of saving a life that is brought about by the treatment—as, for example, by the use of busulfan,[43] immunosuppressive drugs, and radiotherapy. This, of course, has not always been the case, and the medical use of two of the drugs (inorganic trivalent arsenic and chlornaphazine) has been abandoned.[44] In other cases the balance of risk and benefit has yet to be fully assessed, and the use of the agent is continued under controlled conditions in the hope that the benefit will prove to outweigh the long-term harm. (This is more acceptable with medicines than with many other putative carcinogens, for the risks and benefits of particular medical practices usually affect the same individual.)

Some of the agents listed above that continue to be used are used in the treatment of relatively uncommon conditions, and the sum of the cancers caused can amount to no more than a few hundred throughout the entire country each year. Three, however, are used extensively: *a*) ionizing radiations, *b*) estrogens, and *c*) steroid contraceptives.

a) Ionizing radiations.—These are sometimes essential for treatment and are often essential for diagnosis, the latter use probably accounting for about 85% of the total dose given in the United States. The Interagency Task Force on the Health Effects of Ionizing Radiation (1979) estimated that the dose of radiation currently received by the U.S. population for medical purposes amounts to about 18 million rems/year. On the assumptions that we have made previously (section 5.6), the continuation of present exposure levels would imply the eventual production of about 4,500 fatal cancers a year. Much of the irradiation is, however, received by people with an expectation of life that is too short for any significant chance of developing radiation-induced cancer (because of illness or age), and the total future effect may be no more than half this amount. Past patterns of use of X-rays differ from present usage in many ways, diagnostic examinations in previous decades being less frequent but involving higher doses than is usual today, so the total number of current cancers due to past irradiation may differ from the 2,000 or so per year that will arise from current irradiation. However, an estimate of similar magnitude still seems plausible. To this we must add a small proportion (perhaps 5% or less) of all childhood cancers produced by exposure of the fetus from radiological examination of the mother's abdomen during pregnancy (and perhaps by the liberal use of X-rays in certain intensive care units for premature babies), so that the total proportion of cancers attributable to the medical use of ionizing radiations is probably about one-half of 1%. This number is distressingly large, and any reduction in the frequency of use or the dosage of diagnostic irradiation, especially for fetuses (and perhaps children), might eventually prevent a few hundred cancer deaths per year.

b) Estrogens.—These have been given extensively for the relief of postmenopausal symptoms and the prevention of osteoporosis. The extent to which their use causes cancer is still disputed, but in our view the case for believing that they have been responsible for the recent increase in incidence of endometrial cancer is strong (Jick et al., 1980). How many cases they are continuing to produce throughout the country is difficult to estimate. In some areas they may have been responsible for one-half the cases of endometrial cancer, which in turn accounts for 1% of all cancer deaths. It should be noted, however, that endometrial cancer has a relatively good prognosis, and those cases associated with the use of estrogen a particularly good prognosis, so that the proportion of deaths attributable to the use of the drug must have been a small fraction of 1%, a conclusion reinforced by the continuing steady decline in endometrial cancer death certification rates (but *see* discussion in appendix D of the biases affecting these apparent downward trends). The major uncertainty, however, concerns the role of estrogens in the production of cancer of the breast (Hoover et al., 1976). They are certainly not responsible for more than a small proportion of such cases, but the disease is so common and the fatality rate so high (breast cancer accounts for a total of 9% of all cancer deaths) that the production of even 5% of cases would be important. Whether they

---

[43] The excess risk of leukemia due to busulfan seemed to be restricted to overdosed patients who developed pancytopenia.

[44] As has been the specific use of *a*) one particular estrogen to improve the outcome of pregnancy (diethylstilbestrol), which led to the development of vaginal adenocarcinoma in several hundred young women who were exposed to the drug when a fetus in their mother's abdomen and *b*) two radioactive materials (thorium and thorotrast) that were used, respectively, in the treatment of skeletal disease and as a contrast medium in radiology.

are responsible for any at all is, in our opinion, still awaiting judgment.

c) Oral contraceptives.—Finally, we must consider the steroid contraceptives, known colloquially as "the pill," and taken daily by millions of young women. Since pregnancy at an early age reduces the risk of cancer of the breast in middle and old age, any effective form of contraception (male or female) must increase these risks. We have discussed this effect in our section on reproductive factors and shall not attribute such cancers specifically to the pill. Components of the pill given in much larger doses to laboratory animals have caused cancers of the breast and liver, and there is no doubt of their carcinogenic potential. Hormonal carcinogens are, however, in a class which is different from most other chemical carcinogens, and there is a good case for believing that some of the effects are not proportional to the size of the dose but may be very much less or even non-existent at the low levels that are used to produce contraception. Many studies of women on the pill have been conducted and many are still continuing, and precise quantitative estimates of the risks associated with the use of the different varieties should be available in the course of the next 5 or 10 years. A review of the evidence available up to 1977 was undertaken by an expert committee of the World Health Organization (WHO, 1978), which concluded that there was no certain evidence of an effect on the incidence of cancers of the breast or cervix uteri, but that one type of the pill, the use of which is now abandoned, had probably caused some cases of cancer of the endometrium, and that other types of the pill which are still in use did occasionally cause benign tumors of the liver. These last, though not cancers in the ordinary sense of the word, can cause fatal internal hemorrhage and on very rare occasions indeed give rise to true malignant disease. Conversely, there is some evidence to suggest that the pill may reduce the risk of cancer of the ovary, a common cause of death which may be related to the cyclic activity of the ovary which the pill suppresses. On balance, we have assumed that the total number of cancers currently arising each year from the use of the pill is too small to be taken into account in our calculations, but the evidence needs to be kept under regular review.

Sum of Effects of All Medical Agents or Procedures

In sum, our best estimate of the proportion of cancer attributable to medical practice is about 1%, one-half of which is attributable to irradiation. However, the number of ways in which drugs, especially the chronic use of drugs, might in principle increase or decrease cancer incidence rates is almost limitless, for drugs are used precisely because, in the doses actually given, they cause substantial physiological changes. Consequently, the fact that the known hazards may not add up to more than 1% does not imply that no greater unknown hazards exist. No effective drug can be *guaranteed* to be safe (a message reinforced by the recent clofibrate trial results: Committee of Principal Investigators, 1978) and routine monitoring of the history of prolonged medication of newly diagnosed cancer patients remains essential. The upper confidence limit suggested by early data from the Boston Collaborative Drug Surveillance Program suggests that the percentage of current cancers attributable to long-term drug use, excluding radiation, is 2% (Jick and Smith, 1977), but as more data accumulate this statistical upper limit is likely to decrease.

5.10 Geophysical Factors

Two physical agents present everywhere in the natural world, ionizing radiations and UV light, were among the first factors to be recognized as carcinogenic to humans. UV sunlight is the principal cause of basal cell carcinoma (the so-called "rodent ulcer") of the face and neck in white-skinned people and also causes a high proportion of the squamous carcinomas that occur on parts of the skin that are exposed to the sun. It also contributes to the production of cancer of the lip and melanoma of the skin. Cancer of the lip is becoming much less common as it is also associated with pipe smoking, which has declined in popularity, and those cases that continue to occur seldom cause death if treated soon after the lump appears. Melanoma of the skin, in contrast, is one of those cancers that is increasing most rapidly in white-skinned populations and causes a substantial number of deaths. The incidence of melanoma in different parts of the world correlates fairly closely with the flux of UV light, and xeroderma pigmentosum patients, who cannot repair the damage that UV light does to the DNA of their skin, are at grossly elevated risk of melanoma (Robbins et al., 1974). Although the dose-response relationship is odd, perhaps because regular exposure to sunlight produces a protective suntan, it seems that most cases of melanoma are produced by sunlight. It also seems plausible that the worldwide increase in melanoma among white-skinned people is due, in some part, to the changes in clothing and greater exposure of the skin to sunlight than was customary half a century ago. The relationship is, however, less clear-cut than for basal cell and squamous carcinomas in that the distribution of cases on the surface of the body does not correspond neatly to the degree of exposure. Nor does the increase seem to be limited to melanomas on the exposed areas, although it is greater on these than elsewhere. One explanation could be that sunlight affects the incidence of the disease at sites distant from the irradiated area through hormonal stimulation of melanocytes; another that other and so far unsuspected agents are involved. At this stage we may, perhaps, attribute 90% of lip cancers and 50% or more of melanomas as well as 80% of other skin cancers to UV light (lip cancer in conjunction with smoking), in which case sunlight (especially strong sunlight on white skins) would account for between 1 and 2% of all cancer deaths.

The relationship between cancer and ionizing radiations has been the cause of much debate. Until 30 years ago it was commonly assumed that ionizing radiations of whatever sort (whether X-rays, γ-rays, or α- or β-particles) did not cause cancer unless they were intense enough to cause obvious damage to the irradiated tissue. This, it is now known, is not true and, although there continues to be debate about the exact nature of the dose-response relationship at low doses and about whether α-particles cause relatively more damage for a given amount of ionization than X-rays (because the effects are so much more localized—the so-called "hot spot" effect), most research workers accept that, for the practical purpose of preventing cancer, it may be assumed that at low doses and low dose rates the effect is approximately proportional to the dose. We have elsewhere included estimates of the effect of ionizing radiations in the production of occupational cancer, cancers due to radioactive pollutants, and those due to the use of ionizing radiations for medical purposes. There remains to make an estimate of the effect of cosmic rays and the minute amounts of radon and other radionuclides that occur in the air, in our bodies, and in all natural materials and accumulate inside houses with restricted air exchange. If we assume that each individual receives a whole-body dose of about 100 millirems, the total annual dose received by the whole population will amount to about 22 million rems. [By comparison, the Interagency Task Force on the Health Effects of Ionizing Radiation (1979) estimated that the dose of radiation received by the population from background sources amounts to about 20 million rems/year.] On the assumptions we have made previously (section 5.6), this would imply the production of about 5,500 cancer deaths a year, or 1.4% of the total.

In sum, geophysical factors may account for about 3% of all cancer deaths, and we regard this figure as quite reliably known. However, although 3% are *attributable* to geophysical factors, almost none of the 1.4% attributable to background ionizing radiation are avoidable, nor (given the ubiquity of sunlight) are some of those attributable to UV light. The proportion that might reasonably be described as *avoidable* by practicable means depends on the way in which melanoma risk depends on the exact pattern of exposure to sunlight but is probably only about 1%, and certainly not more than 2%.

5.11 Infection

Infection has often been suspected of being a cause of cancer, but the statistical evidence establishes beyond doubt that cancer is not, in general, an infectious disease in the sense that people who come into close contact with a patient (such as nurses, doctors, and spouses of patients) do not have a higher risk of developing the disease than do others. Reports have occasionally been published of the occurrence of an unusually large number of cases of some rare type of cancer in a small community within a year or so, but such "clusters" must be expected to occur periodically by chance alone in a population as large as that of the United States. Detailed investigation does not suggest that any type of cancer tends to occur in this way, except perhaps for acute lymphocytic leukemia in childhood and Burkitt's lymphoma, and even in these two types of cancer the evidence of clustering is weak.

Viruses

It is possible that viruses capable of transmission from one person to another are important in the development of some types of cancer, but, if they are, it seems likely that they are widespread in the community and that a variety of other factors determine whether or not exposure to the virus leads to the development of disease. If viral infection does produce cancer, it may do so in a variety of ways. One that has been intensively investigated in the last two decades is by becoming integrated into the genetic material of a human stem cell and modifying its behavior in such a way that the cell becomes the parent of a malignant clone. One virus that seems able to do this is the Epstein-Barr virus, which occurs ubiquitously and is the specific cause of glandular fever (infectious mononucleosis). In special circumstances (which are apparently more common in tropical Africa and South China than elsewhere), the virus may insert inself into the DNA of a reticuloendothelial cell or of an epithelial cell in the nasopharynx and perhaps in consequence give rise, respectively, to a Burkitt's lymphoma or a nasopharyngeal carcinoma, all the cells of which are characterized by containing some of the viral DNA in combination with their own. Final proof of the viral etiology of these two types of tumors, however, remains elusive.

No other human cancers have been shown to be characterized by the presence of viral DNA in the genetic material of the cells, but this may be because the methods of detecting the presence of the virus are not sufficiently sensitive. It would not be surprising if viral infection were eventually shown to be an essential factor in the production of various other types of cancer, including cancer of the cervix uteri (on the grounds referred to in section 5.5), cancer of the penis (since the wives of men who develop it have an abnormally high risk of developing cancer of the cervix uteri but not of any other cancer; Graham et al., 1979; Smith et al., 1980), acute lymphatic leukemia in childhood (partly because the disease may recur, affecting the donated cells, after an affected patient has received a marrow transplant from a relative who remains healthy), and reticulosarcoma (because of its occasional appearance shortly after an individual has begun to receive, for the treatment of some other condition, immunosuppressive drugs in doses that are large enough to diminish the body's resistance to viruses).

If all these cancers depended on viral infection, the proportion of cancer deaths attributable to infection would be about 4%. The proportion may, however, be much higher as infection, like diet, may contribute to the production of cancer in a variety of indirect ways. It may, for example, promote the development of cancer by causing tissue necrosis or otherwise stimulating the division of stem cells and so sensitizing them to the action of chemical carcinogens. It is possibly in this way that the hepatitis B virus comes to be associated so often with the development of cancer of the liver and that an attack of infectious mononucleosis may bring about a slight increase in the risk of developing Hodgkin's disease.

Bacteria or Parasites

Infection with bacteria or parasites may contribute to the production of the disease in other ways. We have referred in section 5.3 to the possible role of intestinal bacteria in producing (or destroying) carcinogenic metabolites in the large bowel and of salivary duct bacteria in converting nitrates into nitrites and hence facilitating the formation of N-nitroso compounds in vivo, and bacteria could also contribute directly to the formation of N-nitroso compounds in the stomach and bladder. Bacterial infection associated with the development of chronic bronchitis has been thought to increase the risk of lung cancer in cigarette smokers (Rimington, 1971), possibly by impairing the efficiency of the mechanisms for clearing the bronchi and hence permitting more prolonged contact between inspired carcinogens and the bronchial stem cells. Similarly infection could be one link in the chain that results in the association between ulcerative colitis and colorectal cancer, between schistosomiasis (a parasitic infection that commonly affects the bladder in parts of Africa) and bladder cancer, and between clonorchiasis (a parasitic infection of the liver that is common in parts of China) and cholangiocarcinoma.

Conclusions

The examples we have cited are unlikely to be the only ways in which infection affects the risk of developing cancer, but even if they were, the range of acceptable estimates for its contribution would be large. We would, therefore, suggest a figure of about 10% as a very uncertain best estimate of the proportion of cancer deaths somehow attributable to infection (5% perhaps attributable to the action of viruses and a token figure of 5% to allow for the possible role of other infective agents in determining the conditions under which cancer is produced in vivo). The likely role of infectious agents in the etiology of cancer of the uterine cervix provides a lower limit of at least 1%, but we can at present make no useful guess at the upper limit.

5.12 Unknown Causes

From this review it is evident that the specific causes of many of the common cancers have not been iden-

tified. For several of these, and particularly for cancers of the colon, rectum, stomach, and breast, the evidence suggests that dietary factors are likely to play an important part, and we have made an allowance for such factors in assessing the relative importance of different sources of risk. There are, however, several other cancers which, we suspect, are partly due to extrinsic factors (in the broad sense of the term) but which have not been allocated to any particular group of causes. Two types that we have not taken into account are reported to have increased materially in incidence and mortality: namely, myelomatosis and non-Hodgkin's lymphoma. New diagnostic tools (marrow puncture and serum electrophoresis) have transformed the ease of recognition of the former, and it is difficult to be sure how much (if any) of the recorded increase is real. There are, however, other reasons for thinking that environmental factors are important. In addition to marked international differences, differences have been observed within countries. Within Finland, for example, the incidence rates of myelomatosis in different areas correlate positively and strikingly with various indices of prosperity in those areas (Teppo et al., 1980). Both myelomatosis and non-Hodgkin's lymphoma—which together account for about 5% of all cancer deaths—may be largely due to extrinsic causes that have been omitted. Prostate cancer, which accounts for about 10% of cancer deaths in men, must also be regarded as largely extrinsic in origin because of the gross variation in incidence among different communities (e.g., members of the same ethnic groups living in different countries). Confusion between "latent cancer," diagnosed after pathological examination of the prostate, and clinical cancer, which, if untreated, causes death from spread to other organs, has complicated interpretation of the trends in incidence, and it is uncertain how far the high incidence in the United States (and, in particular, in the black population) should be regarded as due to newly introduced agents. The prostate itself is an accessory sex gland under hormonal control, and hormonal secretions, influenced perhaps to some extent by sexual behavior, may be major determinants of the disease. Cancer of another sex organ (the testis, accounting for 0.4% of cancer deaths in men) has also become more common during the past half century. The increase, which was first evident in Denmark (Clemmesen, 1968), now appears to have ceased, and no acceptable explanation for it has been suggested.

Two categories of environmental factors that we have ignored (and may therefore be classed with "unknown factors") are that of psychological stress and that of some form of breakdown of immunological control, both of which have been suggested at intervals throughout this century to play some part in the production of cancer. It is possible, of course, that psychological factors could have some effect, e.g., by modulating hormonal secretions, but we know of no good evidence that they do nor that they affect the incidence of cancer in any other way, except insofar as they lead people to smoke, drink, overeat, or enjoy some other harmful habit. In this respect it is perhaps relevant that studies of patients in mental hospitals provide no evidence of unexpected risks (Clemmesen and Hjalgrim-Jensen, 1977; Baldwin, 1979). Likewise, it might perhaps be that some form of immunological surveillance normally controls the development of certain types of cancer so that failure of such control would affect the onset rate of such cancers and that environmental factors affect the likelihood of such failure, but for the present this is all too speculative to quantify, as is the suggestion that some non-specific generalized effects of "aging" may be relevant.

6. SUMMARY AND CONCLUSIONS

Trends

Examination of the trends in American mortality from cancer over the last decade provides no reason to suppose that any major new hazards were introduced in the preceding decades, other than the well-recognized hazard of cigarette smoking, which has extended from men to women, and the cause (whatever it may be) of the increase in melanoma. Among people over 65 years of age there are increases in *recorded* mortality (especially among the very old) from brain tumors and from some other types of tumor which are not mainly due to smoking, but these apparent increases among the old may chiefly reflect progressive improvements in the accuracy with which the causes of death of old people are recorded (appendix C) due not only to better medical technology but also, in large part, to better medical care for the elderly. Among people under 65 years of age, most of the trends in recorded mortality are downward, those for adults under the age of 45 being particularly favorable, which bodes well for the future. Some decreases are due to improved treatment (for example, in the case of Hodgkin's disease) while some are for unknown reasons (as in the case of cancer of the stomach) but cannot be accounted for by improvements in the outcome of treatment.

Trends in *recorded* incidence rates (in which both fatal and non-fatal cases of cancer are counted) are difficult to interpret because of the difficulty of allowing for the effects of more complete registration and of more screening. The latter is liable to create spurious increases due to the classification as cancer of borderline cases, some of which would never have presented as clinical cancer within the subject's lifetime (as, for example, has probably happened in the case of cancer of the prostate or breast). These difficulties are substantial when we compare recorded cancer incidence rates now with those a quarter of a century ago in particular registries, and other difficulties of noncomparability appear to affect the comparison of the Second National Cancer Survey (1947/8) and Third National Cancer Survey (1969–71) with each other or particularly with the SEER program which has succeeded them. For a few of the less common types of

TABLE 20.—*Proportions of cancer deaths attributed to various different factors*

Text section No.	Factor or class of factors	Percent of all cancer deaths	
		Best estimate	Range of acceptable estimates
5.1	Tobacco	30	25–40
5.2	Alcohol	3	2–4
5.3	Diet	35	10–70
5.4	Food additives	<1	−5[a]–2
5.5	Reproductive[b] and sexual behaviour	7	1–13
5.6	Occupation	4	2–8
5.7	Pollution	2	<1–5
5.8	Industrial products	<1	<1–2
5.9	Medicines and medical procedures	1	0.5–3
5.10	Geophysical factors[c]	3	2–4
5.11	Infection	10 ?	1–?
5.12	Unknown	?	?

[a] Allowing for a possibly protective effect of antioxidants and other preservatives.
[b] *See* section 5.5 for intended meaning.
[c] Only about 1%, not 3%, could reasonably be described as "avoidable" (*see* text). Geophysical factors also cause a much greater proportion of non-fatal cancers (up to 30% of all cancers, depending on ethnic mix and latitude) because of the importance of UV light in causing the relatively non-fatal basal cell and squamous cell carcinomas of sunlight-exposed skin.

cancer, large improvements in curability have occurred, and it is reasonable to hope that improvements will be demonstrated for breast cancer and perhaps for certain other common types of cancer as well. However, the apparent moderate improvements in 5-year relative survival rates over the past quarter of a century are, of course, themselves in part an artifact due to the same changes (in the completeness of case registration and in the nature of the lesions that are diagnosed) that have affected recorded incidence data. Consequently, as we are not convinced that changes in treatment have materially affected the outcome of most of the major types of potentially fatal cancer, it seems to us wiser for most types of cancer to estimate the real trends in disease onset rates chiefly from the recorded trends in mortality since 1950 among people under the age of 65. However, we look forward to the time when the SEER program will provide a sufficiently long and uniform series of data for trends in incidence to be assessed independently of mortality.

The fact that lung cancer rates in the United States, in comparison with those in other countries, are, if anything, somewhat *lower* than might be expected simply on the basis of the number of cigarettes Americans consume (appendix E) and the lack of any apparent overall upward trends in cancer other than those due to tobacco do not, of course, guarantee that apart from tobacco all is well. Indeed, although some thousands of Americans every year are now dying of asbestos-induced cancer, this public health disaster cannot be clearly seen in the national trends (except perhaps for the still rare asbestos-induced mesothelio-mas), so an analysis of trends is clearly a crude tool. We have dwelt on it at length merely because so many people mistakenly believe most cancer onset rates to be rising rapidly and because that belief may in turn be a cause of mistaken priorities in cancer prevention.

Current Causes

The estimates of risk attributable to different classes of environmental agents that we made in section 5 are brought together in table 20. The sum of the estimates is less than 100% despite the fact that some agents interact with one another to produce the disease in the way described in section 4.4. When this happens, the removal of either factor may have almost as much effect as the removal of both so that a few avoidable cancers are counted twice. The sum would, however, have been a good deal more than 100% if it had been possible to characterize the unknown factors referred to in section 5.12. The firmest estimates in table 20 relate to the effects of tobacco, alcohol, and geophysical factors, while by far the largest estimates relate to tobacco and diet.

Similar but less detailed sets of estimates which have been made previously by Wynder and Gori (1977) and by Higginson and Muir (1979) are summarized in table 21.[45] Both sets refer to cases rather than to deaths and hence attribute larger proportions to sunlight than does table 20, and Higginson and Muir refer to "life-style" rather than to diet, meaning by it, however, factors "such as lack of dietary fiber, excess fat and caloric intake, and possibly hormone carcinogenesis." Despite these differences, the patterns described in the three sets of estimates resemble one another reasonably closely, except that we have preferred not to try to force the total to add up to 100%.

Tobacco

Returning to our table 20, the only cause whose effects are both large and reliably known is tobacco, which in 1978 accounted for about 120,000 cancer deaths and which will probably account for between 130,000 and 140,000 U.S. cancer deaths in 1981. Although it appears inevitable that the percentage of U.S. cancer deaths due to tobacco will continue to rise for at

---

[45] We know of no other explicit sets of estimates with which our table 20 can be compared directly. In particular, we know of no formal attempt to make quantitative estimates of the contribution of different causes which embodies the common belief that the majority of cases of cancer could be prevented by the stringent control of chemical pollution of air, food, water, and of occupational exposure. Epstein's popularization of this belief (1978, 1979, 1981b) has been dealt with elsewhere (section 4.1 and Peto, 1980). Finally, although the review of epidemiological knowledge by Maclure and MacMahon (1980) overlaps considerably with our subject matter (and with our conclusions), it does not contain explicit numerical estimates.

TABLE 21.—*Proportions of cancer cases attributed to various different factors by other authors*

Factor or class of factors	Percent of all cancer cases in:			
	England, Birmingham region, based on Higginson and Muir (1979)		United States, based on Wynder and Gori (1977)[a]	
	Male	Female	Male	Female
Tobacco	30	7	28	8
Tobacco/alcohol	5	3	4	1
Diet	—	—	40	57
Life-style	30	63	—	—
Occupation	6	2	4	2
Sunlight	10	10 ⎱	8	8
Ionizing radiations	1	1 ⎰		
Iatrogenic	1	1	—	—
Exogenous hormones	—	—	—	4
Congenital	2	2 ⎱	16	20
Unknown	15	11 ⎰		

[a] Deduced from histograms. Non-environmental factors equated with congenital and unknown.

least a few more years, reaching about 33% by the mid-1980's, non-prohibitive legislation (and the other sources of changes in public awareness discussed in section 5.1) may materially reduce national cigarette usage, while changes to lower tar cigarettes can materially reduce the risk per cigarette. Because the likelihood of such changes cannot be foreseen, longer term prediction of the percentage of U.S. cancer deaths ascribable to tobacco is not reliable. These estimates of the effects of smoking are subject to some small uncertainty because there may be some misdiagnosis of lung cancers as other cancers and vice versa and also because of the need to generalize from the experience of samples of the non-smoking population (whose diet, occupation, and socioeconomic status may not be typical of the country as a whole) in order to estimate the small number ($\approx$12,000) of lung cancers not due to tobacco which must be subtracted from the large number ($\approx$100,000) of U.S. deaths attributed each year to cancer of the lung. Both qualifications are well recognized. Neither affects the validity of the conclusion that smoking is a cause of a large proportion of all cancer deaths, which is based on massive evidence from many sources. They do mean that it is impossible to be sure of the exact attributable risk. However, the current figure cannot be less than 25% or more than 40%. Cigarette smoking also causes many deaths from causes other than cancer, so there are unlikely to be any substantial hidden dangers in its avoidance. The most important area of uncertainty, which could be addressed by the large case–control study of lung cancer which we have recommended, concerns the relative effects of the various low-tar and other types of cigarette. If, as we suspect, the hazards of *long*-term use of low-tar cigarettes are smaller relative to high-tar cigarettes than is suggested by the report of the Surgeon General (1981), this might be of great public health significance, yet reliable information remains elusive.

Diet

We have attributed the largest risk to dietary factors for reasons that are discussed in detail in section 5.3. It must be emphasized that the figure chosen is highly speculative and chiefly refers to dietary factors which are not yet reliably identified. Experimental findings and human observation alike provide many indications that dietary factors are of major importance in determining the risk of cancers of the gastrointestinal tract, some cancers of the female sex organs, and epithelial cancers in general, but there is as yet little decisive evidence on which firm conclusions can be based. From our review in section 5.3 of various current lines of research into dietary factors, it is probable that the most important would turn out to be not the ingestion of traces of powerful carcinogens or precarcinogens (although these should certainly be guarded against) but rather nutritional factors, ranging from gross aspects of diet to vitamins, trace elements, and other micronutrients which may either enhance *or inhibit* carcinogenesis. (If any minor components of diet do indeed materially *reduce* cancer risks, then their discovery might be of more immediate practical value than the discovery of harmful factors, for prescription may be more rapidly acceptable than proscription.) Several promising hypotheses have been developed sufficiently clearly for them to be tested in practice, and more definite evidence should be obtained within the next decade or two, especially if large, randomly controlled evaluations of certain of the more promising methods of intervention are undertaken. [Bailar's (1979) plea that preventive measures be evaluated by scientific criteria as strict as those for laboratory science has our full support.]

Other Factors

None of the other factors in table 20 can approach the importance of tobacco or the probable importance of diet. One of the larger remaining percentages, however, relates to those aspects of sexual and reproductive behavior that affect the incidence of cancers of the breast, reproductive, and genital organs. The figure cited allows only for the known effects of sexual experience and the favorable effects of pregnancy on the incidence of cancer in women, but it is not impossible that some aspects of sexual behavior also affect the risk of cancer of the prostate and perhaps of the testis in men by, for example, infection or modification of hormonal secretion. For males, however, other determinants of hormonal status may be more important, and in the absence of clear leads the reasons for the variation in the incidence of specifically male cancers have been classed here as "unknown." It cannot, of course, be expected that sexual behavior and reproduction will be much influenced by knowledge that they are likely to affect the incidence of cancer

decades hence. When, however, we have more detailed knowledge of the ways in which the various diseases are produced, it may prove possible to diminish the risks by preventing infection, stimulating or inhibiting hormonal secretion, or modifying its effects.

The proportion of cancers that we have attributed to the specific hazards of occupation, pollution, the use of industrial products, medicines, and medical procedures are individually small. That does not, of course, imply that some of them are not of immense importance to sections of the population on whom the risks are concentrated, but it does mean that their control will have relatively little effect on the total incidence of cancer in the whole country. The uncertainties in our estimates have been emphasized, and a large case–control study of lung cancer could greatly reduce the uncertainty in the proportion of cancers currently ascribable to occupational factors in particular as well as perhaps identifying and therefore controlling more rapidly than might otherwise be the case some hitherto unrecognized occupational hazards. Once recognized, occupational hazards can usually be reduced or eliminated by immediately practicable means, which makes their identification particularly valuable. It is odd that despite the resources that are currently being devoted to laboratory tests of chemicals and regulation of occupational factors so little effort is being made to observe in a systematic way what is actually happening to the large numbers of people who might be at risk.

Future Causes

Our estimates of the small proportions of current cancer mortality due to occupation, pollution, etc. relate, of course, chiefly to those factors for which it has been possible to secure some direct evidence of an effect on humans. Many substances have begun to be used in recent years that are mutagenic to bacteria and carcinogenic in one or more species of laboratory animals. How far exposure to these substances will contribute to the production of cancer in humans in the future is a matter for speculation. On general biological principles, which we have discussed in section 4.2, it must be assumed that some (though not all) of these substances will involve a risk of cancer and, even though the doses to which humans are exposed are commonly minute in comparison with those used in laboratory experiments, this is not always the case and some harmful effects must be anticipated.

Cancer in humans is seldom produced until 10 to 20 years after exposure to the carcinogenic agent begins, and even then the risk may be extremely small in comparison with what it would be if exposure were to continue for several more decades. The human evidence that is currently available does not allow us to express any confident opinion about the extent of the harm that the introduction of these substances may or may not do in the future. The trends that are being recorded do not, however, suggest that the United States (or Britain: *see* Doll, 1979b) is beginning to experience an epidemic of cancer due to new factors.

Indeed, were it not for the effects of tobacco, total U.S. death rates would be decreasing substantially more rapidly than they already are, and we are more encouraged by the benefits that are already being demonstrated from the control of known causes of cancer and other disease than we are dismayed by the appearance of new ones.

The intelligent use of laboratory tests should provide a powerful means for the prevention of new hazards in the future. It will, however, be difficult to use them confidently until we have more exact knowledge of the mechanisms of human carcinogenesis and of the various different classes of factors which can accelerate or retard these mechanisms. Reliable quantitative prediction of human risks from animal or other tests is not yet practicable and may not become so for several years yet. However, the use of particular tests to establish approximate priorities for action on the few agents which by that test seem most dangerous (as discussed in section 4.2) may already be practicable, as should the establishment of a routine large-scale ongoing case-control study (presumably through the SEER program) on lung and perhaps some other type(s) of cancer. Such a study would provide objective data on new and old occupational hazards, on the relative effects of various supposedly less hazardous cigarettes, on "passive" smoking, and on trends in lung cancer among non-smokers.

Future Role of Epidemiology

The one trouble with any such studies is that the questions they answer are only those already posited. It may be no bad thing to answer these, but it should be obvious from our review of current lines of research (especially, perhaps, with respect to dietary factors) how far current cancer research may be from even knowing the right questions to ask. The present need, therefore, is for circumstances that will favor inquiry into all sorts of future questions without present knowledge of what these questions will be.

One useful recent development has been the establishment of a U.S. National Death Index, which greatly facilitates the task of the epidemiologist who wishes to ascertain the dates and causes of death of particular groups of people. Such a facility should be conveniently available to all bona fide medical research workers (both in clinical trials and in epidemiology), should not be dependent on financial support from each separate state, and, if possible, should be extended back to at least 1968 to allow assessment of the relevance of smoking, dietary, reproductive or, especially, occupational circumstances that have been recorded in earlier decades. Safeguards for citizens' privacy are understandably becoming increasingly stringent, but in any legislation or discussions of ethical matters special provision should be considered to exempt from restriction the legitimate needs of bona fide medical research workers for confidential access to causes of death (and medical records of non-fatal illnesses) of named individuals, and for confidential access to data on occupation, residence, and exposure to medical agents. (See, for example, the report of the Subcommittee on Oversight and Investigations, 1980.) Such facilities have long been in use in Britain and Scandinavia, and we know of no example of any serious abuse resulting from this provision of data for epidemiological purposes.

Another large step toward facilitating the quick epidemiological testing of novel hypotheses would be the establishment for public use by bona fide medical research workers of a "bank" of blood and perhaps other biological samples[46] (and open-ended questionnaires[47]) from at least a few hundred thousand apparently healthy people whose names would be linked to the National Death Index. Small aliquots of the blood of people dead from one particular cause could then be sold off to research workers (together with aliquots of control samples) for quick case–control studies. The freedom of speculative epidemiologic inquiry that this facility could confer might well transform the epidemiologic study of both neoplastic and non-neoplastic causes of death. Many such banks of specimens already exist, some of which are too small, some of which have been underexploited, and some of which have already been very fruitful in totally unexpected directions; however, no large bank of such samples is publicly available for use by all bona fide epidemiologists with the funds to buy small aliquots from it.

We have noted elsewhere (section 4.3) why a chiefly epidemiological approach is necessary for our present limited aim of a quantitative perspective. More generally, however, if we want to identify ways of preventing substantial proportions of cancer, then two main strategies are possible.

---

[46] The ideal would be to obtain (and store, identified but not analyzed) a sample of blood taken from each subject on two occasions separated by perhaps 1 year, so that the within-person variability of any measured quantity can be estimated, for without this any null results of analyses might be difficult to interpret. Each of these samples should be stored in small subsamples that can be individually retrieved without disturbing the remainder of that sample. The number of biologically significant factors that can, with present or future technology, be estimated in stored blood is large. (It already includes smoking, many dietary factors, many medicaments, many latent or clinical diseases, and certain genetic factors, and may soon include several measures of DNA damage.) If practicable without undue extra cost, simultaneous storage of fecal samples might well be of great additional value.

[47] A practicable scheme might be to ask each subject to self-complete an exhaustive questionnaire relating to their normal dietary, smoking and drinking habits, their present and past main occupations and places of residence, reproductive history, all long-term medicaments they are on or have been on, and a few specific extra questions, and then a 7-day dietary diary, the whole questionnaire to be posted back and microfiched (uncoded). As with the blood, so with the microfiches: Small but unpredictable parts would be of great interest in future years to epidemiologists with novel hypotheses to test.

The "mechanistic" strategy tries to understand the biology of cancer and exhaustively tests masses of the chemical, infective, or physical agents to which people are likely to be exposed to determine which are likely to be the causes of the cancers of today or of the future. The "black box" strategy, which has yielded the most important findings thus far, looks at the cancers that people chiefly die of and then looks for populations (defined by country or county of residence, by dietary, drinking, or smoking habits, by religion, occupation, or reproduction, and by many other aspects of people's life-style or environment) which differ in their death rates from these cancers to determine what seem to be the chief manipulable determinants of today's cancers. Both approaches are needed, but it is perhaps clear from this report where our sympathies chiefly lie. The epidemiological approach should, of course, be influenced by laboratory discoveries, but the dangers of too great a commitment to a mechanistic approach are obvious, especially since the mechanisms underlying the international and other differences between populations in today's common cancers may not yet be understood. A "black box" approach, although it may be less attractive to a pure scientist, may turn out to be the quickest way to learn how to avoid a significant proportion of those major cancers whose causes still elude us.

REFERENCES

ACHESON ED, GARDNER MJ. The ill effects of asbestos on health. In: Asbestos (Vol 2): Final report of the Advisory Committee. Health and Safety Commission. London: Her Majesty's Stat Off, 1979.

Advisory Committee on the Biological Effects of Ionizing Radiations. The effects on populations of exposure to low levels of ionizing radiations (BEIR III). Washington, D.C.: Natl Acad Sci-Natl Res Council, 1979.

ALAVANJA M, GOLDSTEIN I, SUSSER M. A case control study of gastrointestinal and urinary tract cancer mortality and drinking water chlorination. In: Jolley RL, Gorchev H, Hamilton DH Jr, eds. Water chlorination environmental impact and health effects. Vol 2. Ann Arbor, Mich.: Ann Arbor Science, 1978:395-409.

ALBERT RE, chairman. The Carcinogen Assessment Group's quantitative risk assessment on arsenic. Washington, D.C.: Environmental Protection Agency, 1978.

American Industrial Health Council. A reply to "Estimates of the fraction of cancers in the United States attributable to occupational factors." New York: American Industrial Health Council, 1978.

AMES BN, HOLSTEIN MC, CATHCART R. Lipid peroxidation and oxidative damage to DNA. In: Yagi K, ed. Lipid peroxidation in biology and medicine. New York: Academic Press. In press.

AMES BN, MCCANN J. Validation of the Salmonella test: A reply to Rinkus and Legator. Cancer Res. In press.

Analytical Methods Committee. Determination of the crude fibre in national flour. Analyst 1943; 68:276-278.

ANDERSON HA, LILIG R, DAUM SM, et al. Household-contact asbestos neoplastic risk. Ann NY Acad Sci 1976; 271:311-323.

ARCHER VF, GILLAM JD, WAGONER JK. Respiratory disease mortality among uranium miners. Ann NY Acad Sci 1976; 271:280-293.

ARMSTRONG BK. The role of diet in human carcinogenesis with special reference to endometrial cancer. In: Hiatt HH, Watson JD, Winsten JA, eds. Origins of human cancer. Cold Spring Harbor, N.Y.: Cold Spring Harbor Laboratory, 1977:557-565.

ARMSTRONG B, DOLL R. Bladder cancer mortality in England and Wales in relation to cigarette smoking and saccharin consumption. Br J Prev Soc Med 1974; 28:233-240.

ARMSTRONG BK, DOLL R. Environmental factors and cancer incidence and mortality in different countries, with special reference to dietary practices. Int J Cancer 1975a; 15:617-631.

ARMSTRONG B, DOLL R. Bladder cancer mortality in diabetics in relation to saccharin consumption and smoking habits. Br J Prev Soc Med 1975b; 30:151-157.

ARMSTRONG B, LEA AJ, ADELSTEIN AM, et al. Cancer mortality and saccharin consumption in diabetics. Br J Prev Soc Med 1976; 30: 151-157.

BAILAR JC. The case for cancer prevention. JNCI 1979; 62:727-731.

BALDWIN JA. Schizophrenia and physical disease. Psychol Med 1979; 9:611-618.

BARNES AW. Vinyl chloride and the production of PVC. Proc R Soc Med 1976; 69:277-283.

BARTSCH H, MALAVEILLE C, et al. Bacterial and mammalian mutagenicity tests: Validation and comparative studies on 180 chemicals. In: Montesano R, Bartsch H, Tomatis L, eds. Molecular and cellular aspects of carcinogen screening tests. Lyon: IARC, 1980:179-241.

BERENBLUM I, SHUBIK P. A new quantitative approach to the study of the stages of chemical carcinogenesis in the mouse's skin. Br J Cancer 1947; 1:383-391.

BERENBLUM I, SHUBIK P. The persistence of latent tumour cells induced in the mouse's skin by a single application of 9:10-dimethyl-1:2-benzanthracene. Br J Cancer 1949; 3:384-386.

BINGHAM S, WILLIAMS DR, COLE TJ, et al. Dietary fibre and regional large-bowel cancer mortality in Britain. Br J Cancer 1979; 40:456-463.

BIZE IB, OBERLEY LW, MORRIS HP. Superoxide dismutase and superoxide radical in Morris hepatomas. Cancer Res 1980; 40:3686-3693.

BJELKE E. Dietary vitamin A and human lung cancer. Int J Cancer 1975; 15:561-565.

BJELKE E. Dietary factors and the epidemiology of cancer of the stomach and large bowel. In: Aktuelle Probleme der Klinischen Diätetik, Supplement zu "Aktuelle Ernahrungsmedizin." Stuttgart: George Thieme Verlag, 1978:10-17.

BLOT WJ. Changing patterns of breast cancer among American women. Am J Public Health 1980; 70:832-835.

BLOT WJ, FRAUMENI JF. Arsenical air pollution and lung cancer. Lancet 1975; 2:142-144.

BOYD JT, DOLL R, HILL GB, et al. Mortality from primary tumours of bone in England and Wales, 1961-63. Br J Prev Soc Med 1969; 23:12-22.

BRESLOW N, CHAN CW, DHOM G, et al. Latent carcinoma of prostate at autopsy in seven areas. Int J Cancer 1977; 20:680-688.

BRIDBORD K, DECOUFLE P, FRAUMENI JF, et al. Estimates of the fraction of cancer in the United States related to occupational factors. (Bethesda, Md.: National Cancer Institute, National Institute of Environmental Health Sciences, and National Institute for Occupational Safety and Health, Sept. 15, 1978.) See section 5.6 for details of the context in which this manuscript was released.

BRUCE WR, DION PD, KAKIZOE T, et al. A strategy using short-term assays to identify carcinogens that act in man. Nutr Cancer 1979; 1: 4-7.

BUMB RR, CRUMMETT WB, CUTIE SS, et al. Trace chemistries of fire: A source of chlorinated dioxins. Science 1980; 210:385-390.

BURBANK F, FRAUMENI JF. Synthetic sweetener consumption and bladder cancer trends in the United States. Nature 1970; 227:296-297.

BURBANK F. Patterns in cancer mortality in the United States: 1950-1967, Natl Cancer Inst Monogr 1971; 33:1-594.

Bureau of Cancer Control. Cancer incidence and mortality in New York state (exclusive of New York city). Albany: NY State Dept Health, 1976.

Bureau of the Census. Estimates of coverage of population by sex, race, and age: Demographic analysis. Washington, D.C.: U.S. Govt Print Off, 1974.

Bureau of the Census. Population estimates and projections. Washington, D.C.: U.S. Dept Commerce, 1980 (Publication No. 870, series P-25).

BURKITT D. Related disease—related cause: Lancet 1969; 2:1229-1231.

CAIRNS J. Mutation selection and the natural history of cancer. Nature 1975; 255:197-200.

CAIRNS J. The origin of human cancers. Nature 1981; 289:353-357.

CANTOR KP, HOOVER R, MASON TJ, et al. Associations of cancer mortality with halomethane in drinking water. JNCI 1978; 61:979-985.

CARROLL KK. Experimental evidence of dietary factors and hormone-dependent cancers. Cancer Res 1975; 35:3374-3383.

CARROLL KK. Lipids and carcinogenesis. J Environ Pathol Toxicol 1980; 3:253-271.

CEDERLÖF R, DOLL R, FOWLER B, et al. Air pollution and cancer: Risk assessment methodology and epidemiological evidence. Environ Health Perspect 1978; 22:1-12.

CLEMMESEN J. A doubling of morbidity from testis carcinomas in Copenhagen 1943-62. Acta Pathol Microbiol Scand[A] 1968; 72:348-349.

CLEMMESEN J, HJALGRIM-JENSEN S. On the absence of carcinogenicity to man of phenobarbital. In: Statistical studies in malignant neoplasms. Vol. 5. 1977:38-50.

COLE P. Cancer and occupation: Status and needs of epidemiologic research. Cancer 1977; 39:1788-1791.

COLE P, HOOVER R, FRIEDELL GH. Occupation and cancer of the lower urinary tract. Cancer 1972; 29:1250-1260.

Committee of Principal Investigators. A co-operative trial in the primary prevention of ischaemic heart disease using clofibrate. Br Heart J 1978; 40:1069-1118.

Committee on Prototype Explicit Analyses for Pesticides. Regulating pesticides. Washington, D.C.: Natl Acad Sci, 1980.

Connecticut Cancer Epidemiology Unit—see Heston, Kelly, Meigs, et al., 1979.

CONYBEARE G. Effect of quality and quantity of diet on survival and tumour incidence in outbred Swiss mice. Food Cosmet Toxicol 1980; 18:65-75.

COOK JW, HEWETT CL, HIEGER I. The isolation of a cancer-producing hydrocarbon from coal tar. J Chem Soc 1933; 1:395-405.

COOK JW, HIEGER I, KENNAWAY EL, et al. The production of cancer by pure hydrocarbons. Proc R Soc B 1932; 111 (part I):455-484.

COOK PJ, BURKITT DP. Cancer in Africa. Br Med Bull 1971; 27:14-20.

CRAMER W, The prevention of cancer. Lancet 1934; 1:1-5.

CRAWFORD MD, GARDNER MJ, MORRIS JN. Mortality and hardness of local water supplies. Lancet 1968; 1:827-831.

CRUMP KS, GUESS HA. Drinking water and cancer: Review of recent findings and assessment of risks. Report prepared by Science Research Systems, Ruston, Louisiana, for the Council on Environmental Quality. Washington, D.C., 1980.

CRUSE JP, LEWIN MR, FERULANO GP, et al. Cocarcinogenic effects of dietary cholesterol in experimental colon cancer. Nature 1978; 276:822-824.

CUTLER SJ, YOUNG JL JR, eds. Third National Cancer Survey: Incidence data. Natl Cancer Inst Monogr 1975; 41:1-454.

CUZICK J. Radiation-induced myelomatosis. N Engl J Med 1981; 304:204-210.

DARBY SC, REISSLAND JA. Low levels of ionizing radiations and cancer—are we underestimating the risk? J R Stat Soc A. In press.

DAVIES JM. Stomach cancer mortality in Workshop and other Nottinghamshire mining towns. Br J Cancer 1980; 41:438-445.

DAVIES JM, SOMERVILLE SM, WALLACE DM. Occupational bladder tumour cases identified during ten years' interviewing patients. Br J Urol 1976; 48:561-566.

DAVIS DL, MAGEE BH. Cancer and industrial chemical production. Science 1979; 206:1356-1358.

DEVESA SS, SILVERMAN DT. Cancer incidence and mortality trends in the United States: 1935-74. J Natl Cancer Inst 1978; 60:545-571.

DEVESA SS, SILVERMAN DT. Trends in incidence and mortality in the United States. J Environ Pathol Toxicol 1980; 3:127-155.

DOLL R. Bronchial carcinoma: Incidence and aetiology. Br Med J 1953; 2:521-527 and 585-590.

DOLL R. Cancer and ageing: The epidemiological evidence. Oncology, vol V:1-28, Chicago: Year Book Med Publ 1971.

DOLL R. Strategy for detection of cancer hazards to man. Nature 1977; 265:589-596.

DOLL R. Atmospheric pollution and lung cancer. Environ Health Perspec 1978; 22:23-31.

DOLL R. An epidemiological perspective on the biology of cancer. Cancer Res 1978; 38:3573-3583.

DOLL R. Nutrition and cancer: A Review. Nutr Cancer 1979; 1:35-45.

DOLL R. The pattern of disease in the post-infection era: National trends. Proc R Soc Lond B 1979b; 205:47-61.

DOLL R, GRAY R, HAFNER B, et al. Mortality in relation to smoking: 22 years' observations on female British doctors. Br Med J 1980; 280:967-971.

DOLL R, HILL AB. A study of the aetiology of carcinoma of the lung. Br Med J 1952; 2:1271-1286.

DOLL R, HILL AB, GRAY PG, et al. Lung cancer mortality and the length of cigarette ends: An international comparison. Br Med J 1959; 1:322-325.

DOLL R, PETO R. Mortality in relation to smoking: 20 years' observations on male British doctors. Br Med J 1976; 2:1525-1536.

DOLL R, PETO R. Cigarette smoking and bronchial carcinoma: Dose and time relationships among regular and lifelong non-smokers. J Epidemiol Community Health 1978; 32:303-313.

DORN HF. Increase in cancer of lung. Indust Med 1954; 23:253-257.

DORN WF, CUTLER SJ. Morbidity from cancer in the United States. Public Health Monogr 1955; 29 (parts I, II):1-207.

DUNGAL N, SIGURJONSSON J. Gastric cancer and diet. A pilot study on dietary habits in ten districts differing markedly in respect of mortality from gastric cancer. Br J Cancer 1967; 21:270-276.

DUNN BP, FEE J. Polycyclic aromatic hydrocarbon carcinogens in commercial sea foods. J Fish Res Board Can 1979; 36:1469-1476.

EFRON B, MORRIS C. Stein's paradox in statistics. Sci Am 1977; 236:119-127.

End Results Program. Cancer patient survival. In: Axtell LM, Asire AJ, Myers MH, eds. Bethesda, Md.: National Cancer Institute, 1976 [DHEW publication No. (NIH)77-992].

End Results Program. Trends in survival 1960-63 to 1970-73. In: Myers MH, Hankey BF, eds. Bethesda, Md.: National Cancer Institute, 1976 [DHEW publication No. (NIH)80-2148].

ENSTROM JE. Cancer and total mortality among active Mormons. Cancer 1978; 42:1943-1951.

ENSTROM JE. Rising lung cancer mortality among nonsmokers. JNCI 1979a; 62:755-760.

ENSTROM JE. Cancer mortality among low-risk populations. UCLA Cancer Center Bull 1979b; 6:3-7.

ENSTROM JE. Cancer mortality among Mormons in California during 1968-75. JNCI 1980; 65:1073-1082.

ENSTROM JE, GODLEY FH. Cancer mortality among a representative sample of nonsmokers in the United States during 1966-68. JNCI 1980; 65:1175-1183.

EPSTEIN S. The politics of cancer. San Francisco: Sierra, 1978.

EPSTEIN S. The politics of cancer. Garden City, New York: Anchor Pr./Doubleday, 1979.

EPSTEIN S. Letter to the Editor: Theories of cancer. Nature 1981a; 289:115-116.

EPSTEIN S, SWARTZ JB. Fallacies of lifestyle cancer theories. Nature 1981b; 289:127-130.

FEINLEIB M, SORLIE P, MCGEE D, et al. On a possible inverse relationship between serum cholesterol and cancer mortality in four epidemiological cohorts. Paper read at 53rd annual meeting of the American Epidemiological Society, April 10, 1980.

FINE DH, ROSS D, ROUNBEHLER DP, et al. Formation in vivo of volatile N-nitrosamines in man after ingestion of cooked bacon and spinach. Nature 1977; 265:753-754.

FLETCHER CM, PETO R, TINKER CM, et al. The natural history of chronic bronchitis and emphysema. Oxford: Oxford Univ Press, 1976.

FOOTE CS. Photosensitised oxidation' and singlet oxygen: consequences in biological systems. In: Pryor W, ed. Free radicals in biology. New York: Academic Press, 1976; 2:85-133.

FORBES WF. Intervention in smoking in Canada, with particular reference to economic aspects. Paper presented to WHO expert committee on smoking control, Geneva, 23-28 October, 1978.

Fortune Magazine. The Fortune survey. III. Cigarettes. Fortune 1935 July:11-116.

FOX M. On the diagnosis and treatment of breast cancer. JAMA 1979; 241:489-494.

FOX AJ. Occupational mortality 1970-72. In: Population Trends, Autumn 1977. Office of Population Censuses and Surveys, London: Her Majesty's Stat Off, 1977: 1-8.

FOX AJ, ADELSTEIN AM. Occupational mortality: Work or way of life? J Epidemiol Community Health 1978; 32:73-78.

FRASER P, CHILVERS C, BERAL V, et al. Nitrate and human cancer: A review of the evidence. Int J Epidemiol 1980; 9:3-11.

GARFINKEL L. Cancer mortality in nonsmokers: Prospective study by the American Cancer Society. JNCI 1980; 65:1169-1173.

GARFINKEL L. Time trends in lung cancer mortality among non-smokers and a note on passive smoking. JNCI 1981; 66:1061-1066.

GASKILL SP, McGUIRE WL, OSBORNE CK, et al. Breast cancer mortality and diet in the United States. Cancer Res 1979; 39:3628-3637.

GÄSTRIN G. Programme to encourage self-examination of breast cancer. Br Med J 1980; 1:193.

General Household Survey. General household survey for 1976. Office of population censuses and surveys. London: Her Majesty's Stat Off, 1978.

GERMAN J. The cancers in chromosome-breakage syndromes. In: Okada S, et al., eds. Proceedings of 6th International Congress of Radiation Research. Tokyo: Japan Assoc Radiation Research, Univ Tokyo, 1979.

GESAMP [IMCO/FAO/UNESCO/WMO/IAEA/UN Joint Group of Experts on the Scientific Aspects of Marine Pollution (GESAMP)]. Impact of oil on the marine environment. Report No. 6, Stud GESAMP, 1977.

GOODALL CM, FOSTER JH, FRASER J. Fluoridation and cancer mortality in New Zealand. NZ Med J 1980; 92:164-167.

GORI G, BOCK F, eds. Banbury report No. 3: A safe cigarette? Cold Spring Harbor, N.Y.: Cold Spring Harbor Laboratory, 1980:1-364.

GRAHAM S, PRIORE R, GRAHAM M, et al. Genital cancer in wives of penile cancer patients. Cancer 1979; 44:1870-1874.

GRIFFIN AC. Role of selenium in the chemoprevention of cancer. Adv Cancer Res 1979; 29:419-442.

GUESS H, CRUMP K, PETO R. Uncertainty estimates for low-dose-rate extrapolations of animal carcinogenicity data. Cancer Res 1977; 37: 3475-3483.

HAENSZEL W. Studies of migrant populations. J Chronic Dis 1970; 23:289-291.

HAENSZEL W, LOVELAND DB, SIRKEN MG. Lung-cancer mortality as related to residence and smoking histories. I. White males. J Natl Cancer Inst 1962; 28:947-1001.

HAMMOND EC, GARFINKEL L, SEIDMAN H, et al. Some recent findings concerning cigarette smoking. In: Hiatt HH, Watson JD, Winsten JA, eds. Origins of human cancer. Cold Spring Harbor, N.Y.: Cold Spring Harbor Laboratory, 1977:101-112.

HAMMOND EC, GARFINKEL L. General air pollution and cancer in the United States. Prev Med 1980; 9:206-211.

HAMMOND EC. Smoking in relation to the death rates of one million men and women. In: Epidemiological study of cancer and other chronic diseases. Natl Cancer Inst Monogr 1966; 19:127-204.

HAMMOND EC, SEIDMAN H. Smoking and cancer in the United States. Prev Med 1980; 9:169-173.

HAMMOND EC, SELIKOFF IJ, LAWTHER PL, et al. Inhalation of benz-pyrene and cancer in man. Ann NY Acad Sci 1976; 271:116-124.

HAMMOND EC, SELIKOFF IJ, SEIDMAN H. Asbestos exposure, cigarette smoking and death rates. Ann NY Acad Sci 1979; 330:473-490.

HARRIS CC. A delayed complication of cancer therapy—cancer. JNCI 1979; 63:275-277.

HARDELL L, ERIKSSON M, LENNER P, et al. Malignant lymphoma and exposure to chemicals, especially organic solvents, chlorophenols and phenoxy acids: a case-control study. Br J Cancer 1981; 43:169-176.

HARSANYI Z, GRANEK IA, MACKENZIE DW. Genetic damage induced by ethyl alcohol in *aspergillus nidulans*. Mutat Res 1977; 48:51-74.

HEASMAN MA, LIPWORTH L. Accuracy of certification of cause of death, General Register Office, Studies on Medical & Population Subjects, No. 20, Her Majesty's Stat Off, London: 1966.

HENDERSON B, PETO J. Manuscript in preparation.

HENNEKENS CH, SPEIZER FE, ROSHER B, et al. Use of permanent hair dyes and cancer among registered nurses. Lancet 1979; 1:1390-1393.

HERITY B, MORIARTY M, BOURKE GJ, DALY L. A case-control study of head and neck cancer in the Republic of Ireland. Br J Cancer 1981; 43:177-182.

HESTON JF, KELLY JB, MEIGS JW, et al. Forty years of cancer incidence in Connecticut: 1935-1974 (April 1978 tape). Privately available from: Connecticut Cancer Epidemiology Unit, New Haven, Conn., 1979.

HIGGINSON J. Perspectives and future developments in research on environmental carcinogenesis. In: Griffin AC, Shaw AC, eds. Carcinogens: Identification and Mechanisms of Action. New York: Raven Press, 1979.

HIGGINSON J, MUIR CS. Détermination de l'importance des facteurs environmentaux dans le cancer humain: Rôle de l'épidémiologie. Bull Cancer (Paris) 1977; 64:365-384.

HIGGINSON J, MUIR CS. Environmental carcinogenesis: Misconceptions and limitations to cancer control. JNCI 1979; 63:1291-1298.

HILL MJ, HAWKSWORTH GM, TATTERSALL G. Bacteria, nitrosamines and cancer of the stomach. Br J Cancer 1973; 28:562-567.

HINDS MW. Mesothelioma in the United States. J Soc Occup Med 1978; 20:469-471.

HIRAYAMA T. Diet and cancer. Nutr Cancer 1979; 1:67-81.

HIRAYAMA T. Non-smoking wives of heavy smokers have a higher risk of lung cancer: A study from Japan. Br Med J 1981; 282:183-185.

HOGAN MD, HOEL DG. Estimated cancer risk associated with occupational asbestos exposure. Risk Analysis. In press.

HOGAN MD, CHI P-Y, HOEL DG, MITCHELL TJ. Association between chloroform levels in finished drinking water supplies and various site-specific cancer mortality rates. J Environ Toxicol Pathol 1979; 2:873-887.

HOLLSTEIN MJ, McCANN J, ANGELOSANTO FA, et al. Short-term tests for carcinogens and mutagens. Mutat Res 1979; 65:133-226.

HOOVER R, GRAY LA, COLE P, et al. Menopause estrogens and breast cancer. N Engl J Med 1976; 295:401-405.

HOOVER R, et al. Progress report to the Food and Drug Administration from the National Cancer Institute concerning the national bladder cancer study. NCI, 1980. Unpublished. See also Lancet 1980; 1:837-840.

HOWE GR, BURCH JD, MILLER AB, et al. Artificial sweeteners and human bladder cancer. Lancet 1977; 2:578-581.

Interagency Task Force on the Health Effects of Ionizing Radiation. Final Report. In: Libassi FP, chairman. Washington, D.C.: 1979.

International Agency for Research on Cancer. Cancer incidence in five continents (Vol. III). In: Waterhouse J, Muir C, Correa P, et al., eds. IARC Sci Publ 1976; 3:1-584.

International Agency for Research on Cancer. Long-term and short-term screening assays for carcinogens: A critical appraisal. IARC Monogr 1980; suppl 2:1-426.

IARC Intestinal Microecology Group. Dietary fibre, transit-time, fecal bacteria, steroids, and colon cancer in two Scandinavian populations. Lancet 1977; 2:207-211.

IARC Working Group. An evaluation of chemicals and industrial processes associated with cancer in humans based on human and animal data: IARC monographs volumes 1 to 20. Cancer Res 1980; 40:1-12.

International Union Against Cancer. Cancer incidence in five continents. In: Doll R, Payne P, Waterhouse J, eds. UICC technical report. Berlin: Springer-Verlag, 1966.

International Union Against Cancer. Cancer incidence in five continents. Vol. II. In: Doll R, Muir CS, Waterhouse JA, eds. Geneva: International Union Against Cancer, 1970.

JABLON S, BAILAR JC III. The contribution of ionizing radiation to cancer mortality in the United States. Prev Med 1980; 9:219-226.

JICK H, SMITH PG. Regularly used drugs and cancer. In: Hiatt HH, Watson JD, Winsten JA, eds. Origins of human cancer. Cold Spring Harbor, NY: Cold Spring Harbor Laboratory, 1977.

JICK H, WALKER AM, ROTHMAN KJ. The epidemic of endometrial cancer: A commentary. Am J Public Health 1980; 70:264-267.

JICK H, WALKER AM, SPRIET-POURRA C. Post-marketing follow-up. J Am Med Assoc 1979; 242:2310-2314.

JOSE DG. Dietary deficiency of protein amino-acids and total calories on development and growth of cancer. Nutr Cancer 1979; 1:58-63.

KAHN HA. The Dorn study of smoking and mortality among U.S. veterans: Report on eight and one-half years of observation. Natl Cancer Inst Monogr 1966; 19:1-125.

KANAREK MS, CONFORTI PM, JACKSON LA, et al. Asbestos in drinking water and cancer incidence in the San Francisco Bay area. Am J Epidemiol 1980; 112:54-72.

KARK JD, SMITH AH, HAMES CG. The relationship of serum cholesterol to the incidence of cancer in Evans County, Georgia. J Chronic Dis 1980; 33:311-322.

KARK JD, SMITH AH, SWITZER BR, HAMES CG. Serum vitamin A (retinol) and cancer incidence in Evans County, Georgia. JNCI 1981; 66:7-16.

KESSLER II. Cancer mortality among diabetics. J Natl Cancer Inst 1970; 44:673-686.

KESSLER II, CLARK JP. Saccharin, cyclamate, and human bladder cancer. No evidence of an association. JAMA 1978; 240:349-355.

KING H, LOCKE FB. American white Protestant clergy as a low-risk population for mortality research. JNCI 1980a; 65:1115-1124.

KING H, LOCKE FB. Cancer mortality among Chinese in the United States. JNCI 1980b; 65:1141-1148.

KING PJ. An assessment of the potential carcinogenic hazard of petroleum hydrocarbons in the marine environment. Rapports et Procedes Verbales 1977; 171:202-211.

KINLEN LJ, HARRIS R, GARROD A, et al. Use of hair dyes by patients with breast cancer: A case-control study. Br Med J 1977; 2:366-368.

KMET J. The role of migrant populations in studies of selected cancer. J Chronic Dis 1970 23:305-324.

KOLONEL LN. Cancer patterns of four ethnic groups in Hawaii. JNCI 1980; 65:1127-1139.

LABARTHE DR. Methodologic variation in case-control studies of reserpine and breast cancer. J Chronic Dis 1979; 32:95-104.

LANIER AP, BLOT WJ, BENDER TR, et al. Cancer in Alaskan Indians, Eskimos, and Aleuts. JNCI 1980; 65:1157-1159.

LAWTHER PJ, WALLER RE. Trends in urban air pollution in the United Kingdom in relation to lung cancer mortality. Environ Health Perspec 1978; 22:71-73.

LEE AM, FRAUMENI JF JR. Arsenic and respiratory cancer in man: An occupational study. J Natl Cancer Inst 1969; 42:1045-1052.

LEE JA, STRICKLAND D. Malignant melanoma: Social status and outdoor work. Br J Cancer 1980; 41:757-763.

LEE PN. Tobacco consumption in various countries. Research paper No. 6. 4th ed. London: Tobacco Research Council, 1975.

LEE PN. Statistics of smoking in the United Kingdom. Research Paper No. 1. 7th ed. London: Tobacco Research Council, 1976.

LEE PN, GARFINKEL L. Mortality and type of cigarette smoked. J Epidemiol Community Health 1981; 35:16-22.

LEW EA, GARFINKEL L. Variations in mortality by weight among 750,000 men and women. J Chronic Dis 1979; 32:563-576.

LINSELL CA, PEERS FG. Field studies on liver cell cancer. In: Hiatt HH, Watson JD, Winsten JA, eds. Origins of human cancer. Cold Spring Harbor, NY: Cold Spring Harbor Laboratory, 1977:549-556.

LOCKE FB, KING H. Cancer mortality risk among Japanese in the United States. JNCI 1980; 65:1149-1156.

LYON JL, GARDNER JW, WEST DW. Cancer incidence in Mormons and non-Mormons in Utah during 1967-75. JNCI 1980a; 65:1055-1061.

LYON JL, GARDNER JW, WEST DW. Cancer in Utah: Risk by religion and place of residence. JNCI 1980b; 65:1063-1071.

MACLENNAN R, DA COSTA J, DAY NE, et al. Risk factors for lung cancer in Singapore Chinese, a population with high female incidence rates. Int J Cancer 1977; 20:854-860.

MACLURE KM, MACMAHON B. An epidemiological perspective of environmental carcinogenesis. Epidemiol Rev 1980; 2:19-48.

MACMAHON B. Prenatal X-ray exposure and childhood cancer. J Natl Cancer Inst 1962; 28:1173-1191.

MACMAHON B, COLE P, BROWN J. Etiology of human breast cancer: A review. J Natl Cancer Inst 1973; 50:21-42.

McGUINNESS EE, MORGAN RG, LEVISON DA, et al. The effects of long-term feeding of soya flour on the rat pancreas. Scand J Gastroenterol 1980; 14:497-502.

MAGNUS K. Trends in incidence of melanoma in Scandinavia. In: Magnus K. Trends in cancer incidence. New York: Hemisphere Publ, in press.

MARTIN AO, DUNN JK, SIMPSON JL, et al. Cancer mortality in a human isolate. JNCI 1980; 65:1109-1113.

MENCK HR, HENDERSON BE. Occupational differences in rates of lung cancer. J Occup Med 1976; 18:797-801.

MESELSON M, RUSSELL K. Comparisons of carcinogenic and mutagenic potency. In: Hiatt HH, Watson JD, Winsten JA, eds. Origins of human cancer. Cold Spring Harbor, N.Y.: Cold Spring Harbor Laboratory, 1977:1473-1481.

MILHAM S JR. Occupational mortality in Washington State, 1950-1971. Washington, D.C.: U.S. Govt Print Off, 1976 [DHEW publication No. (NIOSH)76-175].

MILLER EC, MILLER JA. Naturally occurring carcinogens that may be present in foods. In: Neuberger A, Jukes TH, eds. Biochemistry

of nutrition IA. Baltimore: University Park Pres, 1979 and in Int Rev Biochem 1979; 27:123-165.

Ministry of Agriculture, Fisheries and Food. Survey of vinyl chloride content of polyvinyl chloride for food contact and of foods. Food Surveillance Paper No. 2. London: Her Majesty's Stat Off, 1978.

Ministry of Agriculture, Fisheries and Food. Survey of mycotoxins in the United Kingdom. Food Surveillance Paper No. 4, 1980. London: Her Majesty's Stat Off.

MIRVISH SS, WALLCAVE L, EAGEN M, et al. Ascorbic-nitrite reaction: Possible means of blocking the formation of carcinogenic N-nitroso compounds. Science 1972; 177:65-68.

MODAN B, BARELL V, LUBIN F, et al. Low-fiber intake as an etiologic factor in cancer of the colon. J Natl Cancer Inst 1975; 55:15-18.

MORRISON AS, BURING JE. Artificial sweeteners and cancer of the lower urinary tract. N Engl J Med 1980; 302:537-541.

MUIR CS. 'Classification'. In: Doll R, Muir C, Waterhouse J, eds. Cancer incidence in five continents. IARC Sci Publ 1976; 3:15-23.

National Academy of Science. Drinking water and health (Safe Drinking Water Committee). Washington, D.C.: Natl Acad Sci, 1977.

National Academy of Sciences—see Committee on Prototype Explicit Analyses for Pesticides, 1980.

National Research Council. Halocarbons: Effects on stratospheric ozone (Panel on Atmospheric Chemistry, Assembly of Mathematics and Physical Sciences). Washington D.C.: Natl Acad Sci, 1976.

National Research Council. Nitrates: An environmental assessment (Panel on Nitrates of the Coordinating Committee for Scientific and Technical Assessment of Environmental Pollutants). Washington, D.C.: Natl Acad Sci, 1978.

New York State Department of Health—see Bureau of Cancer Control, 1976.

OBE G, RISTOW H. Mutagenic, cancerogenic and teratogenic effects of alcohol. Mutat Res 1979; 65:229-259.

Occupational Safety and Health Administration. Inflationary impact statement. Washington, D.C.: U.S. Dept Labor, 1976.

Occupational Safety and Health Administration. Estimates of the fraction of cancer in the United States related to occupational factors—see Bridbord et al., 1978.

OETTLÉ AG. Cigarette smoking as the major cause of lung cancer. S Afr Med J 1963; 37:935-941, 958-962, 983-986.

Office of Technology Assessment, United States Congress. Cancer testing technology and saccharin. Washington, D.C.: U.S. Govt Print Off, 1977.

Office of Technology Assessment, United States Congress. Technologies for determining cancer risks from the environment. Washington, D.C.: U.S. Govt Print Off, 1981.

OWEN TB. Tar and nicotine in US cigarettes: Trends over the past twenty years. In: Wynder EL, Hoffman D, Gori GB, eds. Proceedings of the 3d World Conference on Smoking and Health. Modifying the risk for the smoker. Vol. 1. Washington, D.C.: U.S. Govt Print Off, 1976:73-80 [DHEW publication No. (NIH)76-1221].

PACKER JE, MAHOOD JS, MORA-ARELLANO VO, et al. Free radicals and singlet oxygen scavengers. Biochem Biophys Res Comm 1981; 98: 901-906.

PAMUKCU AM, YALCINER S, HATCHER JF, et al. Quercetin, a rat intestinal and bladder carcinogen present in bracken fern (Pteridium aquilinum). Cancer Res 1980; 40:3468-3472.

PEDERSEN E, HOGETUEIT AC, ANDERSON A. Cancer of respiratory organs among workers at a nickel refinery in Norway. Int J Cancer 1973; 12:32-41.

PERCY C, STANEK E, GLOECKLER L. Accuracy of cancer death certificates and its effect on cancer mortality statistics. Am J Public Health 1981; 71:242-250.

PETO J. Genetic predisposition to cancer. Banbury report 4—Cancer incidence in defined populations. Cold Spring Harbor, NY: Cold Spring Harbor Laboratory, 1980:203-213.

PETO R, ROE FJ, LEE PN, et al. Cancer and ageing in mice and men. Br J Cancer 1975; 32:411-425.

PETO R. Epidemiology, multistage models, and short-term mutagenicity tests. In: Hiatt HH, Watson JD, Winsten JA, eds. Origins of human cancer. Cold Spring Harbor, NY: Cold Spring Harbor Laboratory, 1977:1403-1428.

PETO R. Cancer Risk. New Sci 1977b; 73:480.

PETO R. Clinical Trial Methodology. Biomedicine (special issue) 1978; 28:24-36.

PETO R. Detection of risk of cancer to man. Proc R Soc Lond [Biol] 1979; 205:111–120.

PETO R. Distorting the epidemiology of cancer: The need for a more balanced overview. Nature 1980; 284:297–300.

PETO R, DOLL R, BUCKLEY JD, et al. Can dietary beta-carotene materially reduce human cancer rates? Nature 1981; 290:201–208.

PETRAKIS NL. Some preliminary observations on the influence of genetic admixture on cancer incidence in American Negroes. Int J Cancer 1971; 7:256–258.

PHILLIPS RL. Role of life style and dietary habits in risk of cancer among Seventh Day Adventists. Cancer Res 1975; 35:3515–3522.

PHILLIPS RL, GARFINKEL L, KUZMA JW, et al. Mortality among California Seventh Day Adventists for selected cancer sites. JNCI 1980; 65:1097–1107.

PIKE MC, GORDON RJ, HENDERSON BE, et al. Air pollution. In: Fraumeni JF, ed. Persons at high risk of cancer: An approach to cancer etiology and control. New York: Academic Press, 1975:225–238.

PIKE MC, JING JS, ROSARIO IP, et al. Occupation: "Explanation" of an apparent air pollution related localized excess of lung cancer in Los Angeles County. In: Whittemore AS, Breslow NE, eds. Energy and health. Philadelphia: Society for Industrial and Applied Mathematics, 1979:3–15.

PINTO SS, ENTERLINE PE, HENDERSON V, et al. Mortality experience in relation to a measure of arsenic trioxide exposure. Environ Health Perspec 1977; 19:127–130.

POLLACK ES, HORM JM. Trends in cancer incidence and mortality in the United States, 1969–76. JNCI 1980; 64:1091–1103.

POTT P. Chirurgical observations relative to the cataract, polypus of the nose, the cancer of the scrotum, the different kinds of ruptures and the mortification of the toes and feet. London, 1775.

PURCHASE IF. Inter-species comparisons of carcinogenicity. Br J Cancer 1980; 41:454–468.

REDDY BS, COHEN LA, MCCOY D, et al. Nutrition and its relationship to cancer. Adv Cancer Res 1980a; 32:237–345.

REDDY JK, AZARNOFF DL, HIGNITE CE. Hypolipidaemic hepatic peroxisome proliferators form a novel class of chemical carcinogens. Nature 1980b; 283:397–398.

Registrar General for England and Wales. Occupational mortality 1970–72: Decennial supplement. London: Her Majesty's Stat Off, 1978.

RIMINGTON J. Smoking, chronic bronchitis, and lung cancer. Br Med J 1971; 2:373–375.

ROBBINS JH, KRAEMER KH, LUTZNER MA, et al. Xeroderma pigmentosum: An inherited disease with sun sensitivity, multiple cutaneous neoplasms and abnormal DNA repair. Ann Intern Med 1974; 80:221–248.

ROE FJ, TUCKER MJ. Recent developments in the design of carcinogenicity tests on laboratory animals. Proc Europ Soc for the Study of Drug Toxicity 1974; 15:171.

ROE FJ. Are nutritionists worried by the epidemic of tumours in laboratory animals? Proc Nutr Soc 1981; 40:57–65.

ROGOT E, MURRAY JL. Smoking and causes of death among U.S. veterans: 16 years of observation. Public Health Rep 1980; 95:213–222.

ROSE G, SHIPLEY MJ. Plasma lipids and mortality: A source of error. Lancet 1980; 1:523–525.

ROTHMAN K, KELLER R. The effect of joint exposure of alcohol and tobacco on risk of cancer of the mouth and pharynx. J Chronic Dis 1972; 25:711–716.

ROUS P, KIDD JG. Conditional neoplasms and sub-threshold neoplastic states: Study of tar tumours of rabbits. J Exp Med 1941; 73:365–389.

RUSSELL B. Introduction to history of Western philosophy. London: George Allen & Unwin, 1946.

SAFFIOTTI V, MONTESANO R, SELLAKUMAR AR, et al. Experimental cancer of the lung. Inhibition by vitamin A of the induction of tracheo-bronchial squamous metaplasia and squamous cell tumors. Cancer 1967; 20:857–864.

SARACCI R. Asbestos and lung cancer: An analysis of the epidemiological evidence on the asbestos-smoking interaction. Int J Cancer 1977; 20:323–331.

SCHNEIDERMAN MA. NCI statement before the Subcommittee on Health and Scientific Research of the Senate Committee on Human Resources. 5 March, 1979.

SCHNEIDERMAN MA. "What's happening to cancer in our advanced industrial society? Have the risks been overstated?" Presented at the Conference on Epidemiological Methods for Occupational and Environmental Studies, Washington, D.C., 3–5 December, 1979.

SCHNEIDERMAN MA. Calculations cited by Toxic Substances Strategy Committee, 1980 (160–166) and in Science 1980; 209:998–1002.

SCHRAUZER GN, ISHMAEL D. Effects of selenium and of arsenic on the genesis of spontaneous mammary tumors in inbred C3H mice. Ann Clin Lab Sci 1974; 4:441–447.

SCHRAUZER GN, WHITE DA, SCHNEIDER CJ. Cancer mortality correlation studies—III: Statistical associations with dietary selenium intakes. Bioinorg Chem 1977; 7:23–31.

Second National Cancer Survey, 1947/8 (SNCS)—see Dorn and Cutler, 1955.

SELIKOFF IJ, LILIS R, NICHOLSON WJ. Asbestos disease in United States shipyards. Ann NY Acad Sci 1979; 330:295–311.

SELIKOFF IJ, SEIDMAN H. Cancer of the pancreas among asbestos insulation workers. Paper read at the International Meeting on Pancreatic Cancer, Louisiana State University, New Orleans, 10 March, 1980.

SHAMBERGER RJ, FROST DV. Possible protective effect of selenium against human cancer. Can Med Assoc J 1969; 100:682.

SHAMBERGER RJ. Relationship of selenium to cancer. I. Inhibitory effect of selenium on carcinogenesis. J Natl Cancer Inst 1970; 44:931–936.

SHUBIK P. Food additives, contaminants, and cancer. Prev Med 1980; 9:197–201.

SIEMIATYCKI J, DAY NE, FABRY J, COOPER JA. Discovering carcinogens in the occupational environment: A novel epidemiologic approach. JNCI 1981; 66:217–225.

SLAGA TJ, SIVAK A, BOUTWELL RK, eds. Carcinogenesis—a comprehensive survey. Vol. 2. New York: Raven Press, 1980.

SMITH PG, KINLEN LJ, WHITE GC, et al. Mortality of wives of men dying with cancer of the penis. Br J Cancer 1980; 41:422–428.

SPINGARN NE, SLOCUM LA, WEISBURGER JH. Formation of mutagens in cooked foods. II. Foods with high starch content. Cancer Lett 1980; 9:7–12.

SPORN MB, NEWTON DL. Chemoprevention of cancer with retinoids. Fed Proc 1979; 38:2528–2534.

STENBACK F, PETO R, SHUBIK P. Initiation and promotion at different ages and doses in 2,200 mice. Br J Cancer 1981. In press.

STEWART A, WEBB J, HEWITT D. A survey of childhood malignancies. Br Med J 1958; 1:1495–1508.

STICH HF, STICH W, ROSEN MP, et al. Clastogenic activity of caramel and caramelised sugars. Mutat Res Letters. In press.

Subcommittee on Oversight and Investigations, Committee on Interstate and Commerce. Data Transfer Restrictions Impede Epidemiological Research. (Committee Print 96-IFC 63, 96th Congress, 2d Session) Washington, D.C.: U.S. Govt Print Off, 1980.

SUGIMURA T, NAGAO M, KAWACHI T, et al. Mutagen-carcinogens in food, with special reference to highly mutagenic pyrolytic products in broiled foods. In: Hiatt HH, Watson JD, Winsten JA, eds. Origins of human cancer. pp 1561–1577, Cold Spring Harbor, N.Y.: Cold Spring Harbor Laboratory, 1977.

SUGIMURA T, NAGAO M. Mutagenic factors in cooked foods. CRC Crit Rev Toxicol 1979; 6:189–209.

Surgeon General (1979, 1980, 1981)—see United States Public Health Service.

Surveillance, Epidemiology and End Results Program (SEER). Cancer incidence and mortality in the United States, 1973–1976, Young JL, Asire AJ, Pollack ES, eds. Bethesda, Md.: NCI, 1978 [DHEW publication No. (NIH)78-1837].

Surveillance, Epidemiology and End Results Program (SEER). see Young et al., 1981.

TAGNON I, BLOT WJ, STROUBE RB, et al. Mesothelioma associated with the shipbuilding industry in coastal Virginia. Cancer Res 1980; 40:3875–3879.

TAMURA G, GOLD C, FERRO-LUZZI A, et al. Fecalase: A model for activation of dietary glycosides to mutagens by intestinal flora. Proc Natl Acad Sci USA 1980; 77:4961–4965.

TANNENBAUM A. Initiation and growth of tumors; introduction; effects of underfeeding. Am J Cancer 1940; 38:335–350.

TEPPO L, PUKKALA E, HAKAMA M, et al. Way of life and cancer incidence in Finland. Scand J Soc Med 1980; suppl 19:1-84.

Third National Cancer Survey, 1969-71 (TNCS)—*see* Cutler and Young, 1975.

Toxic Substances Strategy Committee. Toxic chemicals and public protection. Council on Environmental Quality. Washington, D.C.: U.S. Govt Print Off, 1980.

TRICHOPOULOS D, KALANDIDI A, SPARROS L, et al. Lung cancer and passive smoking. Int J Cancer 1981; 27:1-4.

TROWELL H. Ischemic heart disease and dietary fiber. Am J Clin Nutr 1972; 25:926-932.

TUCKER MJ. The effect of long-term food restriction on tumours in rodents. Int J Cancer 1979; 23:803-807.

TURCO RP, WHITTEN RC, POPOFF IG, et al. SST's, nitrogen fertilizer and stratospheric ozone. Nature 1978; 276:805-807.

TUYNS AJ, PÉQUIGNOT G, JENSEN OM. Les cancers de l'oesophage en Ille-et-Villaine en fonction des niveaux de consommation d'alcool et de tabac. Des risques qui se multiplient. Bull Cancer (Paris) 1977; 64:45-60.

United Nations Scientific Committee on the Effects of Atomic Radiation. Sources and effects of ionizing radiation. New York: United Nations, 1977.

U.S. Public Health Service. Smoking and Health. Report of the Advisory Committee to the Surgeon General of the Public Health Service, U.S. Dept. of Health and Human Services, Washington, D.C.: U.S. Govt Print Off, 1964.

U.S. Public Health Service. Smoking and health. A report of the Surgeon General of the Public Health Service, U.S. Dept. of Health and Human Services, Office on Smoking and Health. Washington, D.C.: U.S. Govt Print Off, 1979.

U.S. Public Health Service. Smoking and health. The health consequences of smoking for women. A report of the Surgeon General of the Public Health Service, U.S. Dept. of Health and Human Services, Office on Smoking and Health. Washington, D.C.: U.S. Govt Print Off, 1980.

U.S. Public Health Service. The health consequences of smoking: The changing cigarette. A report of the Surgeon General of the Public Health Service, U.S. Dept. of Health and Human Services, Office on Smoking and Health. Washington, D.C.: U.S. Govt Print Off, 1981.

WAGNER JC, BERRY G, SKIDMORE JW, et al. The effects of the inhalation of asbestos in rats. Br J Cancer 1974; 29:252-269.

WALD N, IDLE M, BOREHAM J, et al. Low serum-vitamin-A and subsequent risk of cancer. Lancet 1980a; ·2:813-818.

WALD N, IDLE M, BOREHAM J, et al. Inhaling habits among smokers of different types of cigarette. Thorax 1980b; 35:925-928.

WALD N, DOLL R, COPELAND G. Trends in the tar, nicotine and carbon monoxide yields of U.K. cigarettes manufactured since 1934. Br Med J 1981; 282:763-765.

WARNER KE. Possible increases in the under-reporting of cigarette consumption. J Am Stat Assoc 1978; 73:314-318.

WATTENBERG LW. Inhibition of chemical carcinogenesis. J Natl Cancer Inst 1978; 60:11-18.

WATTENBERG LW, LOUB WD. Inhibition of polycyclic aromatic hydrocarcon-induced neoplasia by naturally occurring indoles. Cancer Res 1978; 38:1410-1413.

WATTENBERG LW. Inhibitors of chemical carcinogens. J Environ Pathol Toxicol 1980; 3:35-52.

WEST DW, LYON JL, GARDNER JW. Cancer risk factors: An analysis of Utah Mormons and non-Mormons. JNCI 1980; 65:1083-1095.

WILLIAMS RR, STEGENS NL, GOLDSMITH JR. Associations of cancer site and type with occupation and industry from the Third National Cancer Survey Interview. J Natl Cancer Inst 1977; 59: 1147-1185.

WITSCHI H, WILLIAMSON D, LOCK S. Enhancement of urethan tumorigenesis in mouse lung by butylated hydroxytoluene. J Natl Cancer Inst 1977; 58:301-305.

World Health Organization. Prevention of cancer. Geneva: WHO, 1964 (Technical Report Series 276).

World Health Organization. Steroid contraception and the risk of neoplasia. Geneva: WHO, 1978 (Technical Report Series No. 619).

World Health Organization. World health statistics annual: Vital statistics and causes of death, Geneva: WHO, 1977.

World Health Organization. World health statistics annual: Vital statistics and causes of death. Geneva: WHO, 1980.

World Health Organization. WHO. environmental health criteria: Arsenic. Geneva: WHO, In press.

WYNDER EL, BROSS IJ. A study of etiological factors in cancer of the esophagus. Cancer 1961; 14:389-413.

WYNDER EL, GORI GB. Contribution of the environment to cancer incidence: An epidemiologic exercise. J Natl Cancer Inst 1977; 58: 825-832.

WYNDER EL, STELLMAN SD. Artificial sweetener use and bladder cancer. Science, 1980; 207:1214-1216.

WYNDER EL, MUSHINSKI M, STELLMAN S. The epidemiology of the smoker. Proceedings of the 3d World Conference on Smoking and Health. Vol. 1. Washington, D.C.: U.S. Govt Print Off, 1976 [DHEW publication No. (NIH)76-1221].

YAMASAKI E, AMES BN. Concentration of mutagens from urine by adsorption with the non-polar resin XAD-2: Cigarette smokers have mutagenic urine. Proc Natl Acad Sci USA 1977; 74:3555-3559.

YOUNG D. Relationship between cigarette smoking, oral contraceptives and plasma vitamins A, E, C, and plasma triglycerides and cholesterol. Am J Clin Nutr 1976; 29:1216-1221.

YOUNG JL JR, PERCY C, ASIRE A. Surveillance, epidemiology, and end results program: Incidence and mortality data: 1973-1977. J Natl Cancer Inst Monogr 57. In press.

Subsequent correspondence

CLEMMESEN J, NIELSEN A. Morbidity versus mortality. (Letter, with reply by DOLL R, PETO R.) J Natl Cancer Inst 1982; 69:317 & 549-550.

APPENDIX A: AGE STANDARDIZATION PROCEDURES

The age-standardized cancer death certification rates we have utilized are chiefly rates per *100 million* standardized directly to the age distribution of the U.S. 1970 census respondents aged *under 65*, rates per *10 million* standardized to the age distribution of respondents aged *65 or over*, or rates standardized to the age distribution of all 1970 census respondents. The age standardization procedure is described in detail, with an example, as are our reasons for using these unusual denominators, i.e., 100 or 10 million. We have everywhere used age-standardized rates rather than either crude rates or such potentially misleading concepts as "mean latency" or "mean age at diagnosis."

Crude Rates, Age-Specific Rates, and Age-Standardized Rates

Throughout this century in the United States, the total probability of death before age 65 years has been decreasing fairly steadily, and it is now less than half what it was only 50 years ago. Consequently, the percentage of the U.S. population that is over 65 years old has been increasing fairly steadily, and the percentage that is over 75 years old is more than double what is was half a century ago. Throughout the world, old people have probably always been several dozen times more likely to develop cancer in the near future than are young people, and so the increase (due chiefly to the decreases in other causes of death) in the percentage of old people tends to increase the annual percentage of the whole population that will get cancer (i.e., the so-called **crude** total cancer onset rate). This phenomenon is not in itself any cause for alarm—rather the reverse, in fact—but it does mean that we must allow for the steady increase in the proportion of old survivors at high risk of cancer if we wish to use trends in the onset rate of cancer to determine whether the external causes of cancer are more active now than long ago. When we turn our attention from the aggregate of all cancer and examine the many different types of cancer separately, exactly the same applies, of course. The *crude* death rate from each particular type of cancer (total cases in one year divided by total population) not only depends on the onset rate of such cancers among people of a given age, but also depends very strongly on the proportions of the population who are young, middle aged, and old.

Two generally accepted methods of calculating indices of cancer mortality (or, instead, cancer incidence[1]) that are not in expectation materially affected by the age distribution of the population as a whole are to calculate either **age-specific** or **age-standardized** rates, and we have chiefly adopted the latter.

The *age-specific* death rate from some particular type of cancer (e.g., stomach cancer) among some particular population (e.g., U.S. males) is the death rate among the males in some particular narrow range of ages. By convention, the 18 five-year age ranges 0–4, 5–9, 10–14, etc. up to 75–79, 80–84, and finally 85 and over, are usually adopted for the calculation of age-specific death rates.[2] For any one particular type of cancer, separate examination of the variation with time of many of the separate age-specific rates may yield much more understanding than any less detailed analysis would have done. (*See* the discussion of trends in U.S. lung cancer mortality in appendix E for an example of this.) However, we wish to characterize, at least approximately, the current trends in each of several different types of cancer, and tabulation of all the trends in the age-specific rates for each of them would produce such an overwhelming mass of numbers that they would be difficult to grasp, and we have chosen to fall back on the use of age-standardized rates instead.

The *age-standardized* cancer rates that we, together with most other commentators on U.S. national data, have used are then simply defined as a weighted average[3] of the 18 separate age-specific rates. Obviously, the age-standardized rate that we actually calculate by such a procedure depends strongly on which weights we choose to adopt. For example, if we gave positive weights to the first 13 age-specific male stomach cancer death rates (i.e., those for ages 0–4, 5–9, etc. up to 60–64), and zero weights to the last five such rates (65–69, etc.), then we would effectively be ignoring all cancers in people aged 65 or over, and the result might be referred to as "an age-standardized stomach cancer death rate among men *aged under 65*." Conversely, we might do the opposite, giving zero weights to the first 13 age-specific stomach cancer death rates and calculating the age-standardized stomach cancer death rate among men *aged 65 and over*. As a final alternative, we could have done what most other commentators have done and give positive weights to all 18 age-specific

---

[1] Cancer *mortality*, or cancer *death*, rates count only those cancers that cause death (or that directly cause some other disease, such as pneumonia, perhaps, which then causes death), whereas cancer *incidence*, or cancer *onset*, rates count all cases, fatal or not.

[2] Some authors have subdivided the human life-span into decades, or into even longer periods of time, when they calculate age-specific death rates. However, if within some of these large age ranges both the numbers of people at risk and the disease onset rate vary rapidly with age, then the use of such long subdivisions of the human life-span may lead to slight uncertainties of interpretation, especially for those types of cancer such as lung cancer or prostate cancer whose onset rates vary most rapidly with age. By contrast, calculations of the effects of even quite sharp dependencies of both population and disease on age suggest that such difficulties will have no material effects (except, perhaps, in the age range ≥ 85) if the life-span is subdivided into the 18 standard *five*-year age groups.

[3] A weighted average of 18 rates is obtained by first choosing 18 multiplying factors, or "weights"; multiplying each observed cancer rate by its corresponding weight; adding up all these 18 products; and, finally, dividing this total by the total of the 18 weights to obtain the weighted average or age-standardized cancer rate. This procedure is also called "direct age standardization."

rates, yielding an age-standardized cancer death rate that depends to some extent on each of the 18 separate rates.

There are important reasons for examining separately trends in age-standardized mortality at ages above and below 65, because the population estimates are less reliable at older ages, and for many types of cancer errors of death certification at ages over 65 may be so numerous, especially earlier this century, as to distort the apparent trends in the all-ages age-standardized death certification rates quite seriously.

Obviously, age-standardized rates calculated by different authors can be compared directly with each other only if the weights that the different authors have chosen to use are the same, and since most other recent commentators on U.S. cancer onset or death rates seem to have used weights that are proportional to the age distribution of respondents to the U.S. 1970 census (table A1), we have done likewise when we wanted an all-ages standardized death rate. Moreover, when we wanted to calculate age-standardized rates among people aged 65 and over, we have used the last five weights in table A1 for the 5 age groups 65–69, 70–74, 75–79, 80–84, and over 85 (and, of course, zero weights for the first 13 age groups). Likewise, of course, to calculate age-standardized rates among people under age 65, we have used only the first 13 weights in table A1.

In table A2 we give a detailed example of the calculation of our three age-standardized lung cancer death certification rates for U.S. males in 1977. Obviously, the age-standardized rate of 0.31796/thousand males under age 65 could equally well be expressed as 317.96/million or 31,796/100 million. Since there are currently about 100 million American males (and about 100 million females) under age 65, if annual rates for people under 65 are expressed per 100 million, they are numerically of a similar order of magnitude to the annual numbers of cancer. We have therefore presented all our age-standardized cancer rates under age 65 as rates per 100 million, so that they suggest to the reader the approximate annual numbers of cancer deaths involved. Likewise, since there are currently only about 10 million American men (and about 10 million women) aged 65 or over, we have presented all rates among such people as rates per 10 million. Thus we would describe the respective age-standardized rates among men under 65 and among men over 65 that were calculated in table A2 not as 0.31796 and 4.0497/thousand (which misleadingly suggests far fewer cancers among the young), but rather as 31,796/100 million and 40,497/10 million, which correctly suggest the approximate numbers of deaths involved.[4] Readers who

---

[4] Moreover, if these different units are used below age 65 and above age 65, then the all-ages age-standardized rate per 100 million happens to be roughly equal to the sum of the two separate rates, which is a convenient approximation to bear in mind. (Strictly, the all-ages rate per 100 million is 0.901258 times the standardized rate per 100 million at ages 0–64 plus 0.98742 times the standardized rate per 10 million at ages >65.)

would prefer the more usual rates (per thousand or per million) can easily recover them, of course, merely by adjusting the decimal point.

One cannot make valid inferences about increases or decreases in the underlying causes of cancer from examination of trends in the percentage of all deaths attributed to cancer (since this is affected by changes in mortality rates from other diseases), nor from examination of trends in the total number of cancers per year or in the crude cancer rates (because both are affected by purely demographic changes). These propositions are generally accepted by all competent epidemiologists (though not by all propagandists), and we would like to see it equally widely accepted that it is also dangerous to make inferences from trends in overall age-standardized cancer rates if these trends are due chiefly to trends among older people and are not also evident upon examination of the trends in the age-standardized rates among people under age 65. This is not because the deaths of old people are less important, nor because trends among them may be determined by social changes which took place half a century or more ago, but simply because the data on cancer trends among old people are often less reliable. This assertion is documented in subsequent appendices.

Time to Tumor

We have deliberately chosen not to express any of our serious analyses in terms of "latency," "reduced latency," "mean age at onset of tumor," or similar indices, because such concepts and the statistical meth-

TABLE A1.—*Weights used for calculating age-standardized cancer onset rates or death rates (as "weighted averages" of age-specific rates)*

These weights are based on the age distribution of a typical million respondents to the U.S. 1970 census, and so the age-standardized cancer rates that are calculated using these weights are described as "rates standardized to U.S. 1970," or some equivalent phrase.

Age range		Weighting	Sub-total of	Grand total of
No.	Years	factor	weighting factors	weighting factors
1	0–4	84,416		
2	5–9	98,204		
3	10–14	102,304		
4	15–19	93,845		
5	20–24	80,561		
6	25–29	66,320		
7	30–34	56,249	901,258 (<65	
8	35–39	54,656	years of age)	
9	40–44	58,958		1,000,000 (all ages)
10	45–49	59,622		
11	50–54	54,643		
12	55–59	49,077		
13	60–64	42,403		
14	65–69	34,406		
15	70–74	26,789		
16	75–79	18,871	98,742 ≥65	
17	80–84	11,241	years of age)	
18	≥85	7,435		

TABLE A2.—Example: *Calculation of age-standardized lung[a] cancer death certification rates among males in 1977*

Age range No.	Age range Years	No. of 1977 male deaths certified as being due to lung[a] cancer at indicated ages[b]	Estimated[c] male population in indicated age range in mid-1977 (thousands)	Annual age-specific male lung[a] cancer death certification rates/1000	Weight (based on U.S. 1970 census; see table A1)	Product: age-specific rate × weight	Annual age-standardized death certification rate/1000
1	0–4	2	8,090	0.0002	84416	21	—
2	5–9	5	9,051	0.0006	98204	54	—
3	10–14	2	9,922	0.0002	102304	21	—
4	15–19	10	10,896	0.0009	93845	86	—
5	20–24	24	10,404	0.0023	80561	186	—
6	25–29	55	9,378	0.0059	66320	389	—
7	30–34	147	8,016	0.0183	56249	1032	—
8	35–39	423	6,397	0.0661	54656	3614	—
9	40–44	1,119	5,740	0.1949	58958	11494	—
10	45–49	2,921	5,879	0.4969	59622	29623	—
11	50–54	5,780	5,863	0.9858	54643	53869	—
12	55–59	8,607	5,425	1.5865	49077	77863	—
13	60–64	11,495	4,500	2.5544	42403	108316	—
14	65–69	12,987	3,704	3.5062	34406	120635	—
15	70–74	11,479	2,592	4.4286	26789	118638	—
16	75–79	7,972	1,648	4.8374	18871	91286	—
17	80–84	4,241	1,018	4.1660	11241	46830	—
18	≥85	2,038	674	3.0237	7435	22481	—
1–13	0–64	30,590	99,561	—	901258	286568	0.31796[d]
14–18	>65	38,717	9,636	—	98742	399871	4.0497[d]
1–18	All ages	69,307[e]	109,197[e]	—	1000000	686439	0.6864[d]

[a] In this example, we have included not only lung but also all other respiratory tract cancers except larynx.

[b] Excludes 5 men certified as dying of such cancers (*see* footnote a) but with their age at death not known, and probably also excludes well over 5,000 who actually died of lung cancer but were certified as having died of some other type of cancer, of "cancer, site not known," or even of some cause other than cancer. Conversely, various other fatal diseases (especially other cancers that spread to the lungs) may be miscertified as lung cancer. The likelihood of both types of error is greater among men aged ≥65 yr than among younger men.

[c] The population estimates that we used differ from those used by most other authors, in that we have included members of the armed forces serving overseas (because we thought that those developing fatal cancer were likely to return home and be numbered among American deaths) and, more importantly, in that we have used population estimates which have been corrected for census undercount (Bureau of the Census, personal communication; *see* appendix B). In most decennial censuses, a few percent of American whites and *ten to twenty* percent of American non-whites either do not appear at all on census returns or appear with misreported age. If such people were to die of lung cancer their deaths would be included in the numerators of the age-specific rates, so they should also appear in the denominators. Corrected population estimates, however, were available to us only from 1950, so from 1933–49 we have, perforce, used the standard (uncorrected) population estimates.

[d] Total of products divided by total of weights.

[e] The *crude* death rate is 69,307/109,197, or 0.63/1,000.

ods that they engender often yield conclusions that are seriously misleading and rarely (if ever) yield important insights which are not available from examination of the age-specific and age-standardized rates. The reasons for this are discussed in some detail in Appendix 3 to the statistical annex to IARC (1980). *Note* particularly that although arguments based on the supposed effects of carcinogens on tumor latency may suggest that the determinants of particular types of cancer in middle and old age may be very different, we see no good reason to believe this (once temporary cohort effects have been ironed out by the passage of time, in the manner described for lung cancer in appendix E).

APPENDIX B: POPULATION ESTIMATION FOR CALCULATION OF AGE-SPECIFIC RATES

Even in the United States as a whole, the available population estimates (whether or not corrected for census undercount) seem surprisingly unreliable, especially at age 65 and over or especially for non-whites. In the particular areas covered by cancer registries, the uncertainties in estimates of the population at risk may perhaps be even larger. The population estimates we have used for 1950-78 include, wherever possible, both members of the armed forces stationed overseas and people who did not complete their previous decennial census. (Published corrections for "census undercount" require some ad hoc modification for 1950-59.)

Ideally, one would like to use as a denominator for the calculation of age-specific rates all the people who if they had developed cancer would have been counted in the numerator of our rates. For mortality, this ideal denominator includes all people abroad (such as Americans on vacation or business, or members of the armed forces abroad) who would return home and die in the United States if they were to develop cancer. It excludes visitors or legal or illegal immigrants in the United

States who would leave America if they were dying, but it includes those of them who would not and who would get into the National Center for Health Statistics publications if they died. Clearly, the decennial census is a crude tool for estimation of appropriate denominators, especially since a few percent of whites and 10 or 20% of non-whites are unregistered in any given census. Also, many people (especially non-whites) seem to have their age described incorrectly by the person who completes the census return for the household they live in, so that the U.S. Bureau of the Census' own estimates of the percentage undercount vary markedly with age and color in a manner that is not even constant from census to census (text-fig. B1). "Adjustment" of the crude census figures for the "estimated" degree of undercount is necessary, but the available estimates of census undercount are so large, especially for non-whites, and depend so erratically on age that it is difficult to trust either the unadjusted or the adjusted data for non-whites (especially since various different methods of estimation of the degree of undercount considered by the Bureau of the Census, 1974, yielded discrepant results). Also, the "adjusted" estimates for the 1950's that have been published by the Bureau of the Census are strikingly inconsistent with the unpublished adjusted estimates for the 1960's which the Bureau of the Census provided for us (unless there really was a sudden 50% increase in the number of

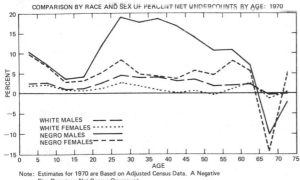

COMPARISON BY RACE AND SEX OF PERCENT NET UNDERCOUNTS BY AGE: 1970

Note: Estimates for 1970 are Based on Adjusted Census Data. A Negative Sign Denotes a Net Census Overcount.

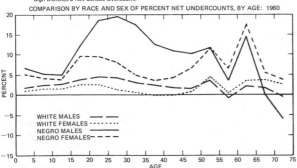

COMPARISON BY RACE AND SEX OF PERCENT NET UNDERCOUNTS, BY AGE: 1960

Note: A Negative Sign Denotes a Net Census Overcount.

TEXT-FIGURE B1.—Comparison of the estimated percentage undercount in the two most recent published U.S. censuses by age and race, showing marked differences (Bureau of the Census, 1974).

males aged 85 and over between 1959 and 1960!).

Moreover, there is no reason to suppose that the dividing line between white and non-white on death certificates used by physicians or state officials when they complete the forms corresponds exactly with the self-completed dividing line between white and non-white on census returns. If there are systematic discrepancies, these will cause systematic errors in the death rates for whites and, particularly, for non-whites If there are time trends in these discrepancies, they will cause artifactual trends in death rates (especially for non-whites) which can be avoided only by pooling both "white" and "non-white" numbers of deaths and population estimates, the ratio of which yields the all-races death rates that we have chiefly used.

We thus require population estimates in each calendar year from 1933 to 1978 (subdivided by sex and age) which include members of the armed forces stationed overseas, which are corrected as accurately as possible for estimated census undercount, and which cover the same states as the annual publication of numbers of deaths (i.e., including Alaska from 1959 and Hawaii from 1960). Such estimates have been constructed (but not published) by the Bureau of the Census for 1960–78 and, by non-comparable methodology, for 1950–59, but not for earlier years. This is unsatisfactory because it means that the absolute numbers of deaths that were tabulated at considerable U.S. government expense each year from 1933 to 1959 cannot be converted easily into death rates that can be compared with modern rates. We therefore relied on the following ad hoc estimates for 1933–59.

1933–39.—We had available to us only estimates that excluded the (then few) members of the armed forces stationed overseas.

1933–49.—We had available to us only estimates that were not corrected for census undercount, which will result in death rates that are a few percent high before 1950.

1959.—Of the available estimates for 1959 that are corrected for census undercount, none include Alaska. Since Alaska contributes only 0.3% of all U.S. deaths, the error can be adequately rectified for 1959 by the use of the corrected population estimates for the contiguous United States in 1959 plus the uncorrected estimate for Alaska in 1960.

1950–59.—Population estimates, corrected for census undercount, have been made available to us by L. Miller, Bureau of the Census, but are increasingly clearly erroneous at ages 75–79, 80–84, and ≥85. On the advice of J. G. Robinson, Bureau of the Census, we took estimates of census undercount on April 1, 1950 and April 1, 1960 among white males age >75,[1]

---

[1] For white males, Robinson estimated 5.31% overcount in 1950 and 0.1% overcount in 1960. For white females, the corresponding figures were 0.90% undercount in 1950 and 4.1% undercount in 1960. For non-white males, they were 13.21% overcount in 1950 and 13.9% overcount in 1960. For non-white females, they were 22.89% undercount in 1950 (!) and 1.0% overcount in 1960.

TABLE B1.—*Population estimates (person-years) used in principal analyses of rates and trends*
Thousands of person-years, corrected for census undercount, including armed forces overseas.

Years[a]	Estimated person-years (thousands) for ages:																	
	0–4	5–9	10–14	15–19	20–24	25–29	30–34	35–39	40–44	45–49	50–54	55–59	60–64	65–69	70–74	75–79	80–84	<85
	White male																	
A	41991	38118	31047	25547	24888	27485	28443	27081	25347	23235	20230	17987	15904	12483	8709	5240	2558	1138
B	45062	42226	38328	31260	25887	25291	27392	28257	26583	24698	22322	18788	16054	13523	9960	6213	3098	1481
C	43390	45397	42502	38619	31596	26235	25396	27166	27821	25815	23644	20819	16758	13556	10691	7070	3722	1860
D	38133	43714	45719	42742	38703	31764	26404	25385	26970	27154	24877	22104	18723	14192	10572	7519	4207	2287
E	34474	38290	43906	45837	42725	38760	31837	26337	25183	26337	26218	23317	20001	15986	11205	7449	4558	2817
F	6620	7312	7993	9148	9026	8204	7224	5885	5026	5067	5182	4933	4105	3388	2436	1541	914	632
	White female																	
A	39989	36315	29660	24559	23965	26608	27925	26725	25186	23343	20579	18823	17118	13935	10445	6855	3749	1880
B	42984	40250	36540	29945	25120	24541	26852	28190	26671	24981	23026	19889	17807	15762	12250	8306	4625	2600
C	41388	43347	40553	36910	30590	25735	24837	26985	28195	26396	24556	22383	18871	16412	13914	9892	5775	3367
D	36317	41729	43692	40904	37359	31099	26062	25043	27048	27944	26007	23842	21417	17437	14497	11335	7072	4511
E	32745	36508	41949	43917	41142	37644	31292	26139	25062	26767	27510	25197	22819	19891	15549	11929	8312	6107
F	6279	6961	7635	8762	8694	7965	7061	5829	5019	5101	5411	5329	4655	4202	3386	2504	1733	1459
	Non-white male																	
A	6826	5578	4494	3865	3636	3649	3832	3626	3270	2735	2410	1931	1432	991	619	354	180	102
B	7906	6877	5666	4557	3911	3725	3717	3725	3325	2991	2562	2124	1673	1199	771	445	221	128
C	8166	7939	6946	5715	4580	3938	3810	3781	3522	3052	2760	2326	1808	1368	922	541	288	156
D	7669	8161	7993	6970	5698	4594	3969	3818	3695	3380	2892	2469	2053	1452	1028	645	342	217
E	7653	7778	8304	8108	7039	5795	4707	4032	3797	3567	3232	2619	2191	1699	1098	706	422	294
F	1536	1584	1607	1697	1575	1336	1062	895	772	741	664	589	431	375	242	148	86	73
	Non-white female																	
A	6759	5515	4444	5841	3603	3610	3656	3328	3098	2653	2392	2013	1599	1180	816	503	322	269
B	7804	6812	5607	4509	3914	3739	3780	3669	3262	3001	2608	2211	1836	1420	974	606	328	271
C	8047	7848	6885	5666	4588	4008	3854	3852	3608	3172	2897	2488	1980	1607	1197	749	415	272
D	7550	8047	7900	6938	5782	4730	4117	3928	3824	3533	3077	2700	2312	1687	1348	964	565	425
E	7482	7674	8175	8042	7168	6085	4951	4238	3966	3763	3475	2910	2537	2059	1407	1069	756	658
F	1499	1557	1583	1677	1593	1406	1130	944	818	783	721	656	510	463	319	217	159	173

[a] A = years 1953–57, B = 1958–62, C = 1963–67, D = 1968–72, E = 1973–77, F = mid-1978 only. The estimated person-years for each 5-year period is the sum of the mid-year populations for the 5 separate years that it spans, and so equals five times the average population in those years.

interpolated linearly between them for July 1, 1950, July 1, 1951, etc. to July 1, 1959, and adjusted the uncorrected 1950–59 census-derived population estimates for white males age 75–79, 80–84 and ≥85 by these interpolated factors. This was repeated separately for white females, for non-white males, and for non-white females.

The population estimates described above are listed in table B1 for 1953–78. Scrutiny of them revealed none of the large-scale resurrection of the dead that is suggested by the uncorrected census-based population estimates that many other analyses of U.S. cancer death rates have utilized.

APPENDIX C: SOURCES OF BIAS IN ESTIMATING TRENDS IN CANCER MORTALITY, INCIDENCE, AND CURABILITY

When assessing either past or current age-standardized rates of cancer incidence or mortality, and particularly when assessing the trends in those rates as we move from the past to the present, certain sources of error must be recognized. For a few cancers, the rates of increase (e.g., lung cancer or melanoma) or decrease (e.g., stomach cancer or cervical cancer) are so large and have continued for so long that it is easy to be sure of their direction and approximate magnitude. However, for most other types of cancer the trends of increase or decrease in their age-specific onset rates over the past decade or two seem much less marked, and it is therefore difficult to estimate these trends reliably. If trends are assessed incautiously, biases in the data may be more important determinants of the apparent trend than the real underlying trends in onset rates will be, which is clearly unsatisfactory. Apart from possible errors in population estimation, which have been discussed in appendix B, there are three main categories of error.

Errors of death certification.—For various reasons, the number of American deaths certified as being due to a particular type of cancer may be substantially in error, especially at age 65 and over or in the years before 1950. For certain types of cancer, however, the best available estimate of the trend in onset rates may be the trend in mortality rates since 1950 among people under age 65.

Errors of incidence registration.—Although incidence data discriminate more reliably between the different types of cancer and are not affected by trends in the curability of particular types, they are affected by the large trends over the last 30 years in the readiness of medical services to register all new cases and (especially recently) by the registration of more and more lumps that are histologically cancer but biologically benign.

Errors of estimation of cure rates.—Estimates of case-fatality rates are subject to many of the same biases that affect estimation of incidence rates, so attempts to correct trends in mortality for trends in curability may in some cases yield less accurate estimates of the trends in real onset rates than the uncorrected trends in mortality might have done.

The origins and effects of these three sources of error are discussed separately below.

Errors of Death Certification

First, cancer patients may die of their cancer without this fact being recognized and may even be certified as having died of some totally different cause, such as pneumonia (for primary or metastatic lung cancer), stroke, senility (for primary or metastatic brain cancer), kidney failure (for myeloma), or some infective disease (for various leukemias or lymphomas). Conversely, patients who did not really die *of* cancer may be miscertified as having done so. In a special enquiry by the British Registrar General into the true causes of some 14,000 deaths in British hospitals in 1959, one-fifth of the deaths thought by the clinician to have been due to cancer were probably due to other causes, whereas a similar number of deaths that the clinicians had not attributed to cancer were probably due to cancer (Heasman and Lipworth, 1966). Many of these clinical errors would not have appeared on death certificates, but many of them would have, and deaths not in hospital might be even less reliably certified than deaths in hospital.

A missed diagnosis of cancer in a dying patient is presumably more likely to occur among old cancer patients than among young ones, if only because the old ones are less likely to be hospitalized. Such errors are likely to have been progressively reduced over the past few decades, particularly in old people since the introduction of Medicare in 1965. We note, for example, that the operation rate in the 10 years after 1965 rose by 45% in men and women age 65 years or over compared with increases of 11 and 17%, respectively, at ages 15–44 years and 45–54 years (National Center for Health Statistics: Unpublished data, and Weiss R: Personal communication). If, as seems likely, fewer diagnoses of fatal cancer are missed nowadays, these changes in medical practice are likely to have caused an artifactual increase in total cancer death certification rates, especially among older people, and the relationship of cancer death certification rates to age

should have been less steep half a century ago than it is today.

Text-figures C1 and C2 show that this is indeed the case, although the effect seems marked only among octogenarians, among whom, if one judges by the shape of the age-incidence graphs in these text-figures, about half of the cancer deaths during the 1930's may have been missed. Alternatively, the population estimates for octogenarians may have been particularly in error, but whatever the reasons artifactual trends in cancer death certification rates are probably more extreme in old age than in middle age. We have therefore examined separately the trends in mortality at ages under 65 (standardized to the age distribution of the U.S. 1970 census respondents under age 65: *See* appendix A) and at older ages (standardized to the older 1970 census respondents).

Second, patients known to be dying with widespread cancer may never have the site of primary origin of their cancer determined, and 6–8% of American cancer death certificates are for "cancer of an unspecified primary site." This percentage is a little lower among whites than among non-whites, and among middle-aged than among older people, but it has not materially changed for decades. Therefore, it may not seriously bias the assessment of trends in cancers of specified sites. However, the 20-odd thousand cancer deaths of an unspecified site each year do represent an uncomfortably large amount of missing information, especially since we do not know, of course, which particular sites have their true death rates most distorted by these exclusions.

Third, patients dying of cancer of one primary site (e.g., lung) may be misdiagnosed as having a cancer originating from another site (e.g., pancreas or brain) if the cancer has either extended itself to other nearby organs or metastasized to distant organs. For example, Boyd et al. (1969), in a special investigation of bone tumor death certificates, concluded that at ages over 65 most so-called "bone tumors" were in fact misdiagnosed secondaries from other sites, and the same may well have been true in the past for liver cancer because bone and liver are not sites where cancers commonly arise, but, along with brain and lung, they are sites to which cancers commonly spread. For Britain in 1959, Heasman and Lipworth (1966) concluded that about one-fifth of the clinical diagnoses of cancer in hospitalized patients specified the wrong site for the primary, and there is no reason to believe that American hospitals were much better (although again it must be noted that not all of these clinical errors would have resulted in incorrect death certificates). Likewise, cancers of one particular cell type may be misdiagnosed as cancers of another cell type; for example, pleural mesotheliomas may be misdiagnosed as ordinary lung cancer or vice versa and myeloid and lymphoid leukemia may be confused with each other, especially in previous decades; all of the different non-Hodgkin's lymphomas may be confused with each other; and malignant and benign fatal brain tumors may be

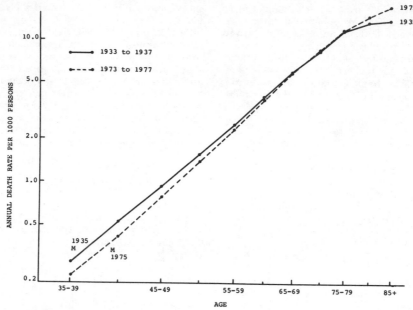

TEXT-FIGURE C1.—Non-respiratory cancer death rates in U.S. males by age, 1935 and 1975 (all races).

confused. There have certainly been substantial changes in the differential diagnosis of the various leukemias and lymphomas, and there may also have been appreciable trends in the differential diagnosis of the various solid tumors, to judge by the fact that in the Second and Third National Cancer Surveys (in 1947/48 and 1969-71) the respective percentages of cancers that were not microscopically confirmed were 26.5 and 9.9%.

Fourth, even if a cancer is correctly diagnosed while the patient is still alive, the correct information may never reach the death certificate. Percy et al. (1981) have tabulated the correspondence between the primary

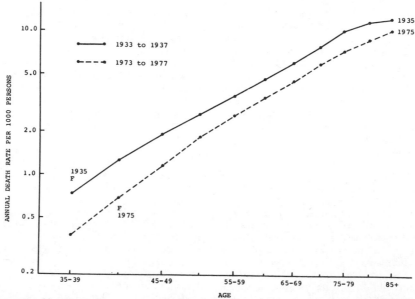

TEXT-FIGURE C2.—Non-respiratory cancer death rates in U.S. females by age, 1935 and 1975 (all races).

site of origin of the cancer, as diagnosed in hospital, and the primary site of origin of cancer, as it eventually appeared on the death certificate, for 82,000 patients in the TNCS. Many discrepancies emerged. Half the cases of rectal cancer were eventually miscertified (chiefly as colon cancer, of course), as were about 20% of all cases of cancer of the lymphoid tissues, buccal cavity, thyroid gland, liver, gallbladder, larynx, cervix and other uterus (the latter two not only as each other), and about 10% of the cases of most other types of cancer. The effects of misdiagnosis and/or miscertification can be circumvented to some extent by adding together into groups the rates for cancers (e.g., all intestinal tumors, all non-Hodgkin's lymphomas, all benign or malignant brain tumors, all leukemias, all lung tumors) that are particularly often confused with each other and also by restricting attention to patients under age 65.

Fifth, treatment may improve sufficiently to have a noticeable effect on total national mortality rates, as has happened over the past decade or two for Hodgkin's disease and for various tumors of uncommon embryomal tissues. (The recent decrease in Hodgkin's disease death rates is, of course, largely or wholly real, and we consider it as a source of "bias" only because we wish to use trends in death rates to indicate trends in onset rates.) The End Results Program (1976, 1980) has estimated the 5-year relative survival rates for various categories of patient, but their method (surveillance of all registered new cancers in one area and of all patients admitted with cancer to certain hospitals in other areas) may be subject to appreciable distortion due to artifactual trends in hospital referral or in the completeness of incidence registration of the nonfatal cases (*see* below). There are thus no wholly reliable data on cancer cure rates. However, it seems safe to conclude that there have been no large increases in the cure rates for the common cancers, so for these the trends in death certification rates may approximate reasonably well to the real trends in real disease onset rates. We shall return to the question of trends in cure rates when we have discussed the artifacts that may affect trends in incidence rates.

Errors of Incidence Registration

Many of the biases listed above that affect cancer death certification rates also affect registered incidence rates, but six additional biases are peculiar to incidence data.

First, population estimation may be more difficult. Our uncertain estimates of the ages and numbers of people in the whole United States were reviewed in appendix B. The uncertainties must presumably be even worse for registry data, where the aim is to count deaths and cases in a defined area (e.g., Detroit, Mich.) with no legal constraints on migration. When is a resident not a resident? The difficulties in estimating the population at risk of getting a cancer that would get registered seem almost as formidable as the problem of registering the cancers. We do not know how

well the population estimates for the SNCS and TNCS really corresponded with the population from whom the registered cases were drawn or whether some of the unexplained discrepancies that we shall discuss between the incidence rates calculated in the 1969–71 TNCS and in the 1973–77 SEER Program derive in part from errors of population estimation.

Second, people only die once and do so at a reasonably well recorded time. By contrast, the symptoms of a cancer may develop gradually, and the patient may attend several medical institutions for diagnostic investigations and treatment, with the age and the spelling of the name varying from one place to another. When all these visits are monitored, it is difficult to arrange a system of record linkage which ensures that this patient gets counted exactly once. Perhaps the problems of mistakenly including the same case twice, or of mistakenly including cases that were first diagnosed before the beginning of the official study period, were worse in earlier years, inflating the cancer onset rates recorded in the 1947/8 SNCS.

Third, standards of diagnosis may improve. A decreasing percentage of cancers (7.3% in the SNCS and only 4.6% in the TNCS) were of liver, bones, or an unspecified site. (This is, of course, a bias that will affect mortality data as well as incidence data.)

Fourth, biases in *registration* rates may be caused by a progressive improvement in the readiness of physicians in the area to collaborate with a cancer registry. For example, Connecticut has maintained one of the best cancer registries in the United States for 45 years, yet table C1 suggests that throughout this period the completeness of their coverage of non-fatal cancers may have been improving so rapidly as to introduce very substantial upward biases into any estimates of trends or of survival rates[1] in those very cancers for which (because an appreciable proportion are curable) registration rates might differ significantly from death certification rates. Likewise, in the Second and Third National Cancer Surveys (in 1947/48 and in 1969–71) the respective proportions of cases that were ascertained by death certificate only, and for which no clinical record was ever found, were 11.2 and 2.2%, suggesting that the earlier survey may have underestimated total incidence rates by about 10%. (*See* footnotes to table C1.)

Fifth, the definition of what constitutes a cancer may change. For example, all salivary gland tumors, whether malignant or of mixed cellularity, were counted up to 1967, but the mixed tumors were dropped thereafter (because their histologic nature was uncertain, but their biologic behavior was usually benign). Likewise, all brain tumors were included in the SNCS, whereas only those specified as malignant were included in the TNCS. This procedure caused a substantial artifactual

---

[1] The cases listed by the Connecticut Cancer Registry comprise nearly half of the material on which the End Results Program (1976, 1980) have estimated trends in cancer cure rates.

TABLE C1.—*Percentages of patients whose cancers were ascertained by death certificate only and for whom no medical details subsequently could be found:[a] Connecticut Cancer Registry, 1935–74[b]*

Years	Cancer							
	Lung		Breast	Prostate	Colon		Pancreas	
	Male	Female	Female	Male	Male	Female	Male	Female
1935–39	32	38	24	39	33	35	46	54
1940–44	28	36	15	23	24	32	30	45
1945–49	24	19	10	15	17	19	32	29
1950–54	17	21	7	12	13	14	24	25
1955–59	15	13	6	9	11	11	21	24
1960–64	8	6	3	5	4	6	9	9
1965–69	2	3	1	2	1	2	4	5
1970–74	2	2	1	1	1	1	2	5

[a] The percentages that would not have been registered but for the death certificate are higher than the percentages cited in this table. (This is because in some instances finding the death certificate may have directed attention to a medical record that would otherwise have been overlooked.) The cited percentages, moreover, are percentages of *all* tumors, fatal or non-fatal, that were ascertained by death certificate only, and so are not as high as the percentage of *fatal* tumors that would not have been registered but for the death certificate. The percentages of non-fatal tumors that were not registered is, of course, not known directly but may also have been large in the earlier years.

[b] Data in tables C1 and C4, and in text-figures C3 to C6, are by courtesy of the Connecticut Cancer Epidemiology Unit (*see* legend to text-fig. C4).

decrease in brain tumor incidence between the two surveys (Devesa and Silverman, 1978). (The distinction between benign brain tumors, brain tumors of unspecified histology, and malignant brain tumors is particularly difficult on death certification data as well because all types may cause death.) Another important change in the opposite direction seems to be an increasing tendency for what would have been called "bladder papillomas" to be termed "carcinomas."

Sixth, one of the most serious sources of error in comparing cancer registration rates in different years stems from the increasingly vigorous search for lumps, because by old age the human body may contain various lumps that, if examined histologically, would be classified as cancer, yet that are biologically so benign that they will not cause any serious symptoms in what life-span remains. For example, by age 70 **2.5%** of males in the areas covered by the TNCS can expect to have been diagnosed as having had prostate cancer (and the annual incidence rate of new cases is only 0.4%, some of which remain quiescent even if treated conservatively), whereas **25%** of the prostate glands of 70-year-old males who die of unrelated causes would, if examined by standard methods, be found to contain "cancer" (Breslow et al., 1977). Likewise, among women undergoing mastectomy for cancer of one breast, and in whom cancer is not already clinically evident in the opposite breast, for many subsequent years **0.5%** per year can expect cancer to become clinically evident in the opposite breast; whereas if the opposite breast is

sampled and examined histologically at the time of the original operation, **15–20%** will already contain "cancer" (Fox, 1979). The scope for biased trends in "incidence" which are due to either more complete registration of what cancers are found or to the finding of "cancers" that would never have caused serious disease is disturbingly large. (A high prevalence of such "incidental" neoplasms is also found in many strains of experimental animals; and even after standardized laboratory autopsy and tissue preparation procedures, animal pathologists often have difficulty agreeing which to call malignant, benign, or merely hyperplastic.)

Comparison of Incidence and Mortality

Trends in total cancer mortality are dominated by the rapid increases in lung cancer, for which (at least since 1950) the differences between incidence and mortality are not important because the case fatality has remained very high. Cancer incidence is dominated by skin cancer, which is in almost all cases so easily cured that many registries do not even attempt to register it. Excluding lung and skin, and excluding people over age 65, we have plotted total U.S. cancer mortality rates 1933–77 against calendar year and compared these with the corresponding total incidence rates in Connecticut (text-fig. C3). The divergence between the two trends is substantial for each sex, and is unlikely to be accounted for by replacement of some fatal type of

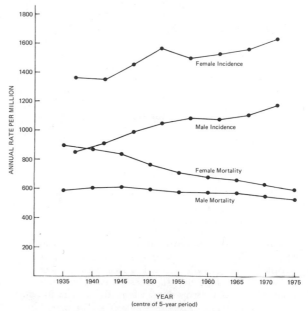

TEXT-FIGURE C3.—Age-standardized certified death rates for entire U.S. population, 1933–77, contrasted with Connecticut registered incidence rates, 1935–74; all cancers except lung and skin. *Rates per million, standardized to the age distribution of all respondents under 65 yr to the U.S. 1970 census, as described in appendix A.*

tumor by a non-fatal type of tumor, by biases in death certification at ages under 65, or by any systematic differences between Connecticut and the United States as a whole. If so, it can be accounted for plausibly only by *a*) improvements in therapy or *b*) biases in incidence registration rates. It seems most unlikely that treatments for the common tumors have improved sufficiently to account for more than a small fraction of the divergences apparent in text-figure C3. (Certainly, the large irregularities in the female incidence data must be artifactual.) The most plausible explanation, therefore, seems that errors in these registered incidence data produce errors in the apparent trends that are much larger than the real underlying trends.

Before accepting this conclusion, however, we shall examine in more detail the trends in mortality and in registered incidence for three particular types of cancer (intestines, breast, and prostate). These three types have been chosen for two reasons: *a*) They are sufficiently common as causes of death to be of substantial public health importance, and *b*) the proportion of diagnosed cases that do not cause death is large enough for differences between incidence and mortality rates to be of substantial interest. (Three other types of cancer—lung, stomach, and pancreas—are also among the six most important causes of death listed in table 1 on page 1197, but for each of these the large majority of diagnosed cases are so rapidly fatal that the differences between incidence and mortality are of less interest.)

Cancer of the intestines.—To render comparable the data on the incidence and mortality of intestinal cancer, we have pooled all intestinal sites, including rectum. (On death certificates, cancers are often described as "intestines, site unspecified," or "large intestine, site unspecified," or "colon, subsite unspecified," a practice that is much less common in the incidence data collected by a good cancer registry. Moreover, there is an increasing tendency not to specify the intestinal subsite on death certificates, and there is substantial nosologic confusion between colon and rectum: *See* appendix D.)

Cancer of the intestines is not difficult to diagnose, even without modern aids, and the surgical treatment of intestinal cancer has not undergone major changes since 1950. To our regret, however, such large discrepancies between the trends in the incidence and in the mortality data were still evident (text-fig. C4) as to suggest the paradoxical conclusion that the rates of change of death certification yield more reliable information about trends in incidence during the 1960's and 1970's than can trends in registered incidence in New York or Connecticut. (Similar discrepancies between trends in registered incidence and trends in certified mortality are, of course, evident among the data for cancer of the female intestines, for which during the past quarter of a century the certified mortality has been decreasing while the registered incidence has been rising. Such discrepancies are also present for cancers of many other sites.)

We have also plotted (text-fig. C4) the data on intestinal cancer incidence provided by the Second National Cancer Survey in 1947/48 (SNCS), by the Third National Cancer Survey in 1969-71 (TNCS), and by the ongoing Surveillance, Epidemiology and End

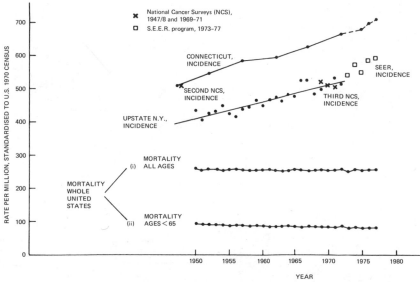

TEXT-FIGURE C4.—Cancer of the intestines (small and large, including rectum): Incidence and mortality in males in the U.S., 1947-77. *Pre-publication access to 1973-77 SEER data (including 1973-77 Connecticut data) to appear in Young et al., 1981, was by courtesy of the Biometry Branch, NCI (E. S. Pollack, Director). Pre-publication access to 1935-74 Connecticut data (April 1978 tape) to appear in Heston et al., 1981, was by courtesy of the Connecticut Cancer Epidemiology Unit (J. W. Meigs, Director). Our other sources of incidence data are New York State Department of Health, 1976, Dorn and Cutler, 1955, and Cutler and Young, 1975.*

Results (SEER) Program in 1973–77, each of which covered about 10% of the U.S. population. Comparison of SNCS with TNCS suggests the same sort of constant incidence as is suggested by the mortality data, and if attention is restricted to ages below 65, a gentle decrease in both mortality (0.4%/yr) and incidence (0.8%/yr) is suggested. By contrast, comparison of the TNCS data with the SEER data suggests a very rapid increase that is even steeper than the one suggested by the longer-term Connecticut and New York data and that is completely incompatible with the gentle and steady long-term decreases in mortality. We are, therefore, unwilling to trust these particular short-term changes in apparent incidence as useful evidence about trends in real cancer onset rates in the 1970's. They may be due in part to more frequent screening for the presence of an intestinal tumor by examination of the feces for small amounts of blood, to the development of colonoscopy as a method of examining the colon, and to the classification of borderline polyps as "malignant" tumors.

Breast cancer.—The trends in age-standardized female breast cancer mortality are almost constant, though very slightly upward. It is likely that these trends are a reasonably accurate reflection of the underlying onset rates of serious breast cancer because the primary treatment of breast cancer (by surgery and/or radiotherapy) did not alter much between the 1950's and the 1970's, while the chemotherapy of early breast cancer was not in common use, and fatal breast cancer is, again, not a difficult disease to diagnose. (During 1968–78 the apparent trends in age-standardized breast cancer mortality have been 0.1% per annum downward among women under age 65 and 0.7% per annum upward among older women, yielding an average of 0.2% per annum upward for all women. *See* appendix D for discussion of possible causes of these small trends in terms of age at first pregnancy, following Blot, 1980.)

By contrast, with the sole exception of the SNCS-TNCS comparison, the available data on breast cancer incidence exhibit bizarre fluctuations from year to year, which are far too large to be ascribable to chance (text-fig. C5). In upstate New York, where a cancer registry has been in operation since 1940, there has been an average increase of about 1% per annum over the past quarter century, a substantial increase which is hardly reflected at all in the mortality data. When the data from the TNCS are compared with those from the SEER Program, wild fluctuations are evident in registered incidence rates during the 1970's that are likewise not reflected at all in the mortality data. These fluctuations can have little or no biological reality and must, in part at least, be determined by fluctuations in public and professional interest, causing many lumps that would not otherwise have been diagnosed as breast cancer to be removed, classified as "locally invasive," and counted among the incidence data. Fox (1979) has already argued that there are numerous breast lumps that are "histologically cancer but biologically benign." To support this argument, Fox noted that although 15–20% of women with cancer in one breast would be found to have "cancer" in the opposite breast if the opposite breast were immediately biopsied, the rate of clinical appearance of cancer in the opposite breast if no biopsy is taken is only 0.5% per year over many subsequent years.

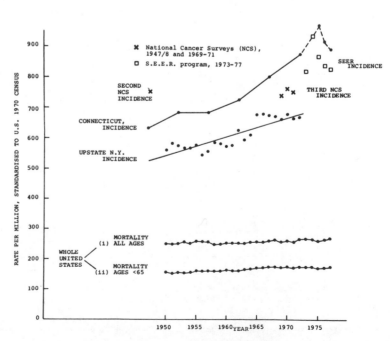

TEXT-FIGURE C5.—Cancer of the breast in females in the U.S.: Incidence and mortality, 1947–77.
For data sources, see text-fig. C4.

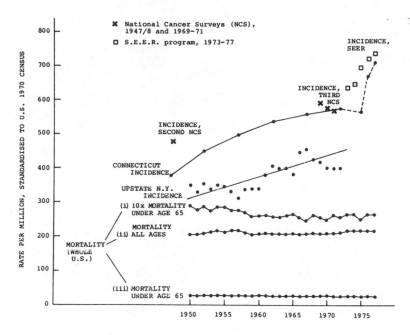

The erratic pattern of variation of the eight data points from TNCS and the SEER Program in text-figure C5 (1969–77) is not explicable by any other obvious source of errors. Although many of the 10 TNCS geographic areas differed from the 10 SEER areas, 4 geographic areas were common to the two studies, and the erratic pattern of the 1969–77 data is virtually unchanged if attention is restricted to these 4 common areas (Pollack and Horm, 1980). Finally, the standard errors on each of these eight points are negligible ($\approx 1.1\%$) compared with the 25% rise in "incidence" recorded between 1971 and 1974.

The same sudden large increases in "incidence," unmatched by any concomitant increases in mortality, were seen in Finland as nationwide breast cancer screening was introduced (Gästrin, 1980). For breast even more than for intestinal cancer, trends in mortality seem much more reliable than trends in incidence, *unless* the trends in incidence are assessed by comparison of the SNCS and TNCS. Comparison of SNCS and TNCS suggests (either by good luck or good management) trends in incidence that are reasonably compatible with the trends in mortality.

Prostate cancer.—Here again, the scope for bias is large, especially since prostate cancer affects the old more than the young to a greater extent than any other cancer. Therefore, prostate cancer incidence (and mortality) trends are especially dependent on the age groups in which both the number of cancers and the estimates of the population at risk are least reliable. A possible great source of difficulty may be that if the prostate glands of men aged 70 who have died of completely unrelated causes, with no clinical history of prostate cancer, are examined post mortem, *1 in 4* (25%) will be found to have "prostate carcinoma" (Breslow et al., 1977). By contrast, by the age of 70 only about 3% of men, even at the SEER incidence rates, will have been diagnosed as having developed clinically evident prostate cancer. (If someone ever invents a method of screening apparently healthy men for prostate cancer, the apparent incidence rates may be expected to rise quickly by several hundred percent!)

Text-figure C6 contrasts the trends in the available incidence data with those in the national mortality data for prostate cancer. It differs from text-figures C4 and C5 in that the mortality data for under age 65 are presented twice, both as they actually are and also multiplied by a factor of 10 merely to make the pattern discernible, because cancer of the prostate gland is an uncommon cause of death before age 65. It also differs from the earlier figures in that, because one-half of all cases of prostate cancer affect men over 75, the uncertainties in the population estimates for the older male age groups in the 1950's cause appreciable irregularities in the all-ages age-standardized rates.

As before, however, the mortality data at ages under 65 suggest no material increase in prostate cancer onset rates; whereas the incidence data collected in Connecticut and New York suggest marked upward trends, and the trend suggested by comparison of the TNCS and SEER data with each other is absurdly incompatible with the mortality data. For prostate cancer, the comparison of the SNCS and TNCS data also suggests some increase in incidence, though an increase that is much more moderate. A moderate increase such as this is compatible with a fairly constant true disease onset rate, slightly biased by progressively more detection as "carcinomas" of biologically benign prostatic neoplasms.

A repeat publication of the SNCS–TNCS comparisons already reported by Devesa and Silverman (1978) but with the data standardized to *a*) U.S. 1970 0-64, *b*) 1970 65+, and *c*) all U.S. 1970 would be useful for many purposes, as would similarly standardized publication of other registry data. (Alternatively, the truncated rates for ages 35-64 recommended in IARC, 1976 would do, and might be better for international purposes.) The age-specific, site-specific data have been published for the total of all areas surveyed in the SNCS and TNCS, and, although they do not allow a comparison to be restricted to the seven areas common to both surveys (or separate examination of melanoma and non-melanoma skin), we have examined the apparent trends among people below 65 years of age in appendix D, table D5, on page 1286.

Errors in Estimation of Cure Rates

We are not chiefly concerned in this report with trends in the treatment of cancer, but rather with trends in the causes of cancer and hence in cancer onset rates. However, since we intend to use trends in cancer mortality as an indication of trends in cancer onset rates, we shall review some of the evidence on trends in cure rates. The most widely accepted data are those reported by the End Results Program (1976, 1980), reviewing the survival of all 169,000 cancer patients registered in Connecticut during 1950–73 and of 284,000 cancer patients seen at a few dozen particular hospitals (mostly in California) over the same period. Despite these large aggregate numbers, some particular types of cancer are so rare that only a few dozen or a few hundred cases are available for study in each period of a few years (e.g., 1950–54 or 1970–73). Omitting all of these rare types except Hodgkin's disease and leukemia, for both of which decreases in the case-fatality rate are so large that random errors are relatively unimportant, we list in table C2 the 5-year relative survival rates observed in certain time periods. There is a general tendency for these survival rates to be slightly better in the 1970's than in the 1950's (e.g., the 5-year relative survival rate recorded for cancer of the female breast has risen from 60% in 1950–54 to 68% in 1970–73). Before this increase can be accepted as evidence for an important improvement in therapy, however, one must ask: What substantial biases might affect the recorded relative survival rates?

First and foremost, many of the biases that we have previously discussed in relation to incidence data might bias the recorded survival rates. In the 1950's, many cases were discovered only via the death certificate, with some earlier medical record then being traced as a result of inquiries initiated because of the death. Such methods clearly underestimate the normal duration of survival in earlier periods. Likewise, in the more recent periods there may have been more breast

TABLE C2.—*Estimated 5-year relative[a] survival percentages among whites: United States, 1950–73*

Type of cancer[b,c]	Patients' sex	Relative survival percentages for patients diagnosed in years:				
		1950–54	1955–59	1960–64	1965–69	1970–73
Stomach	♂	12	12	10	12	12
	♀	11	13	14	14	14
Colon	♂	40	41	42	46	47
	♀	42	47	45	47	50
Rectum	♂	38	39	36	41	43
	♀	43	40	41	45	48
Pancreas	♂	1	1	1	1	2
	♀	2	2	2	2	2
Larynx	♂	52	56	55	63	63
	♀[d]					
Lung	♂	5	7	8	8	9
	♀	9	9	11	13	14
Breast	♀	60	62	64	65	68
	♂[e]					
Cervix uteri	♀	59	60	59	57	64
Endometrium	♀	72	71	73	75	81
Ovary	♀	30	29	34	34	36
Prostate	♂	43	49	52	57	63
Bladder	♂	54	55	58	62	61[f]
	♀	51	56	58	62	60[f]
Kidney	♂	33	36	38	41	44
	♀	34	39	39	43	50
Brain	♂	19	21	20	25	[g]
	♀	22	25	29	33	[g]
Hodgkin's disease	♂	28	36	36	53	66
	♀	34	39	48	57	69
Leukemia[h]		—	—	—	—	—

[a] A *relative* 5-yr survival of 100% would indicate a risk of death no worse than that of the U.S. population as a whole in the relevant time period (matched, of course, for age and sex).

[b] These are the sites for which the End Results Program (1976, 1980) reported on the survival of about 1,000 or more cases/time period, together with Hodgkin's disease and leukemia.

[c] The data refer to all patients diagnosed as having malignant disease of the type specified, irrespective of pathologic stage.

[d] Inadequate data on cancer of the ♀ larynx.

[e] Inadequate data on cancer of the ♂ breast.

[f] Any progressive tendency to class bladder papillomas as bladder carcinomas will produce a progressive but artifactual increase in the relative 5-yr survival rates for bladder "cancer." (*See also* footnote g.)

[g] Changes in the histologic definition of "brain tumor," excluding certain categories of non-malignant tumor, make the reported 5-yr relative survival rates in 1970–73 (♂, 18%; ♀, 22%) difficult to compare with the rates for earlier periods.

[h] Because of recent advances in the treatment of childhood leukemia, it is preferable to examine trends in survival separately for leukemia patients aged <35 yr (≈25% of all leukemia patients).

Year of diagnosis	Leukemia <35 yr: 3-yr relative survival percentage	Leukemia ≥35 yr: 3-yr relative survival percentage
1950–59	5	22
1960–66	10	22
1967–73	24	20

or prostate lumps or bladder papillomas discovered that were considered histologically cancer though being biologically benign, accentuating any upward biases in the trends in curability. Finally, if incurable breast lesions are diagnosed earlier nowadays than in the 1950's, then the 5-year survival may seem better, even if no deaths have actually been delayed. (This last bias may particularly affect breast cancer, but it should not have much effect on most other common cancers which are either completely cured or rapidly fatal.)

Second, patterns of referral to the hospitals collaborating with the End Results Program might alter significantly over a period of a quarter of a century, although it is difficult to predict what the effects of this might be. That this may be so is suggested by the 1-year relative survival rate of 86% for patients with "localized" prostate cancer in 1950–54; surely, 14% of such patients cannot have been killed within a year merely by a localized cancer of the prostate gland, so was their localized prostate cancer diagnosed because of investigation for some life-threatening disease? By 1970–73, the 1-year relative survival for localized prostate cancer had increased to 93%, though the standard therapy (excision and irradiation) had not changed. It is difficult to explain this and to explain the peculiarly large change in 5-year relative survival rates for cancer of the prostate gland as a whole, except in terms of trends in biasing factors.

Because of these various uncertainties, it is a matter of judgment which of the improvements in reported cure rates in table C2 are to be accepted as largely real. The increases over the past quarter century of 5–10% in the 5-year relative survival rates for most of the common cancers (table C2) are very much an extreme upper limit on the amount of improvement which it is plausible to accept, rather than a direct estimate of the actual amount of improvement. The corresponding lower limit on the amount of improvement that it is plausible to accept is zero, and the truth lies somewhere in between. Our view is that the sevenfold improvement in reported leukemia cure rates among people under age 35 must be largely or wholly real (and will probably continue in the late 1970's), as must the twofold improvements in Hodgkin's disease (from one-third relative survival in the 1960's to two-thirds in the early 1970's). However, for many of the common cancers the improvements do not seem to us to be materially larger than bias alone would suggest, and as we do not have evidence for any large improvements in *curative* treatment,[2] we suspect that there has

been substantially less change in case fatality rates than even the 5 or 10% improvements in reported case fatality rates would suggest. Therefore, for most types of cancer the changes in mortality over the past quarter century should certainly be within a few percent, or even less, of the fractional changes in real onset rates.

Conclusion: Which Indicators of Real Trends in Cancer Onset Rates are Most Reliable? *

We have compared trends in mortality with trends in incidence for the few major sites and have found that for those particular sites there are discrepancies too large to be explained plausibly without postulating the existence of serious upward biases in the trends in age-standardization cancer registration rates in both Connecticut and New York since 1950. Similar conclusions would have emerged had we chosen to study certain other sites, and this remains true whether rates of change of incidence and mortality both derive from the same geographic area (table C3) or not (table C4).

By contrast, the trends in onset rates suggested by

TABLE C3.—*Difference between percentage annual rates of change of registered incidence[a] in upstate New York[b] and of certified mortality[a] in upstate New York[b]*

When the difference between these two percentages is positive, which it almost always is, it indicates that registered incidence has been increasing relatively faster than the certified mortality, due perhaps to improvements in therapy during 1960–72 (e.g., for Hodgkin's disease), perhaps to more rapid rectification of biases in registration than of death certification (e.g., for intestines), or perhaps to decreases in overcertification (e.g., liver).

Type of cancer	Annual percentage rate of change of incidence (1950–72) minus annual percentage rate of change of mortality (1960–72)	
	Male	Female
Mouth, pharynx, larynx, or esophagus	0.5	1.7
Lung	1.2	−1.2
Stomach	−0.2	0.0
Intestines	0.9	1.0
Liver	3.2	2.3
Gallbladder	0.5	0.7
Pancreas	1.3	1.2
Melanoma	1.3	0.3
Breast	—	0.6
Bladder	2.4	2.5
Kidney	1.9	1.8
Cervix uteri	—	0.9
Endometrium	—	1.4
Ovary	—	0.9
Prostate	1.6	—
Testis	1.5	—
Brain (malignant only)	1.9	1.5
Leukemia	1.5	1.4
Hodgkin's disease	3.1	1.9

[a] Standardized to U.S. 1970 census, as in appendix A.
[b] Data in this table are from the publication by the Bureau of Cancer Control (1976) of the New York State Department of Health.

---

[2] Even if cancer patients are subdivided into "stages" (e.g., Stage I = no regional or distant spread of the disease, Stage II = regional but not distant, Stage IV = distant spread), no direct assessment of whether therapy has improved can be based on trends in 5-yr survival of patients of a given stage. This is because the steady improvements in the care or technology with which regional or distant disease is sought will, perhaps surprisingly, produce artifactual improvements in prognosis in *each* stage. In Stages I and II this improvement is due to removal of those having micrometastases, whereas in Stage IV it is due to dilution of those having gross metastases by those having micrometastases. Despite these tendencies, the percentage of prostate cancers recorded as "localized" has been increasing over the past quarter century, presumably indicating an increase in the detection as Stage I tumors of lesions that are of borderline significance biologically.

*For discussion of this Conclusion see Clemmesen and Nielsen (1982) and reply.

TABLE C4.—*Incidence trends minus mortality trends*

Annual percentage increase of registered incidence in Connecticut (comparing 1950–54 with 1970–74) minus annual percentage increase in certified mortality in the United States as a whole (comparing 1953–57 with 1973–77). Two comparisons are made, one between trends in incidence and trends in all-ages mortality, the second between trends in incidence and trends in under-age-65 mortality.

Type of cancer, males	Trend in Connecticut minus trends in the rest of United States: Difference[a] between annual percentage rates[b] of change among males	
	Mortality, all ages, vs. incidence, all ages	Mortality, ages <65, vs. incidence, all ages
Mouth, pharynx, larynx, esophagus	−0.4	−1.3
Remaining respiratory (chiefly lung)	−0.1	0.9
Stomach	1.1	0.8
Intestines, including rectum	1.2	1.3
Liver, gallbladder, and bile ducts	0.8	0.8
Pancreas	0.4	0.7
Bladder	2.9	4.1
Kidney	1.1	1.8
Prostate	1.6	1.6
Brain and other parts of the nervous system	0.1	2.0
Leukemia	1.6	2.1
Hodgkin's disease	3.3	3.6
Non-Hodgkin's lymphomas	−0.5	1.3

[a] As in table C3, a positive difference indicates that the annual percentage increase in incidence exceeds that in mortality.
[b] All rates are standardized to the U.S. 1970 census population, as described in appendix A.

comparison of the Second and Third National Cancer Surveys (SNCS and TNCS) with each other do seem more consistent with the concurrent trends in mortality, and so although the registration rate, especially for tumors that are not uniformly fatal, may be subject to various moderate biases,[3] comparison of these two surveys seems a reasonable basis for estimation of the approximate trends in incidence for most solid tumors, except those of the brain and perhaps bladder and

---

[3] Certain such biases might be expected to produce discrepancies between the SNCS-TNCS trends in incidence and the national trends in mortality for those cancers for which neither diagnostic procedures nor cure rates have undergone material change since 1947. Reassuringly, after standardization for age and sex, the 63% decrease in the stomach cancer death rate between 1947 and 1970 was exactly matched by a 64% decrease in the registered incidence rate of stomach cancer between the SNCS and the TNCS. Despite this reassurance, of course, net biases of about 0.5%/yr in either direction could easily exist, with some types of tumor affected differently from others. Unfortunately, the magnitude of this uncertainty is as great as the magnitude of changes which, if real, would be scientifically important.

salivary gland. The comparison of these two surveys has been well presented by Devesa and Silverman (1978; *see* also Devesa and Silverman, 1980), in parallel with a discussion of the concurrent trends in mortality, and we shall not reproduce their detailed tabulations, though a graphic presentation of some of their SNCS-TNCS comparisons appears in text-figs. 5 and 6 on page 1211. Since comparison of the SNCS and TNCS might be slightly more reliable if attention were restricted to ages under 65, and also if "all races" were presented, this comparison is provided in table D5 on page 1286.

The one comparison of incidence rates that seems completely unreliable is that based on the Third National Cancer Survey, 1969–71 (TNCS) and the Surveillance, Epidemiology and End Results (SEER) Program, 1973–77. Quite fantastic and irregular variations in incidence are suggested by such comparisons (either between the two studies or within SEER), ten times greater than could plausibly be attributed to chance, and a hundred times greater than the corresponding annual changes in mortality over the past few decades. Perhaps because some other commentators have not examined the TNCS–SEER trends on the same graphs as the SNCS data and the long-term trends in mortality, our conclusion that the TNCS–SEER trends are unreliable is not widely accepted. Various commentators, among them the Toxic Substances Strategy Committee (TSSC, 1980), in their recent report to the President of the United States, have concluded, *chiefly on the basis of Pollack and Horm's (1980) comparison between TNCS and SEER*, that real cancer incidence rates are increasing rapidly (at 1.3%/yr in males and 2.0%/yr in females). We have given good reasons for distrusting this method for determining incidence trends for the common cancers and see no reason to trust it for the less common cancers. Pollack and Horm (1980) at least express a reasonable degree of caution in their conclusions, but the TSSC does not, and in its main text it generates a firm (and ill-founded, in our view) impression that epidemic increases in cancer are now in progress over and above those attributable to tobacco (appendix E). Anyone who, examining the data in text-figures C4, C5, and C6, can conclude that the most reliable estimate of trends in cancer onset rates is that provided by the TNCS–SEER comparisons deserves a medal for bravery. We have instead preferred to estimate current trends in U.S. cancer onset rates approximately by comparison of the Second and Third National Cancer Surveys, and, more reliably (at least for many of the common cancers), by examination of the trends since 1950 in the age-standardized death rates among people of all races under age 65.

Our argument that "the SNCS-TNCS comparison may be reasonably accurate because it is reasonably consistent with the mortality trends among people under age 65" is, of course, rather circular. After all, if we allow only incidence data that indicate trends exactly identical with the trends in mortality, we might as well not waste time with anything but the mortality data. However, it may be advisable at least to examine both incidence and mortality data, even though the mortality data seem generally more trustworthy. Our tabulations of both, therefore, appear in appendix D.

APPENDIX D: U.S. AGE-STANDARDIZED CANCER DEATH RATES DURING THE PAST FEW DECADES

This appendix presents the detailed data on which the rather general assertions in section 4.1 about trends in cancer mortality during the past few decades were based.

Trends in Total Cancer Mortality Since 1933

After the long list in appendix C of possible biases and difficulties of interpretation, the actual mortality data seem (either refreshingly or deceptively!) simple and straightforward. Table D1 gives trends in age-standardized death certification rates since 1933 (the first year for which all states had to notify the causes of all deaths centrally) for people under 65, and table D2 gives the same trends for older people. The cancer death rates are subdivided into "respiratory" cancer[1] and "non-respiratory" cancer, since the respiratory cancers are dominated by lung cancer and are available as a reasonably consistently defined category throughout 1933–77.

Overall, there are clearly no epidemic increases in mortality from the aggregate of all non-respiratory types of cancer—rather the reverse, in fact—and we discuss the trends in lung cancer mortality in more detail in appendix E. On the basis of appendix E, we conclude that among people under age 65 the increases (and decreases, among younger males) in respiratory cancer death certification rates are mostly real, at least since 1950, and can be largely or wholly[2] accounted for by the effects of cigarette smoking, as long as proper allowance is made for the many decades that elapse between the onset of regular cigarette smoking and its full effects on lung cancer. Contrary to common belief, age-specific total death rates are still improving, and were it not for the substantial ill effects of cigarette smoking (both on respiratory cancer and on the aggregate of all causes of death except neoplasms), Americans would be living in a time of even more rapidly

decreasing age-specific death rates, both in middle age and in old age, than is already the case.

Trends in Site-Specific Cancer Mortality Since the Middle of the Century

It is uncertain how far back trends in American cancer death certification rates can be relied on (and the reliability is different for old and young and for different types of cancer, of course), but 1950 seems a sensible starting point for the estimation of modern trends, at least for the solid tumors. In 1950 there were new rules for coding death certificates, there was a new census (and population estimates corrected for estimated census undercount are available from the Bureau of the Census only from 1950 onward), the classification of cancer had just begun to be based on a reasonably modern International Classification of Diseases (the 6th ICD), so that, for example, Hodgkin's disease was classified as a neoplasm (rather than as an infective disease!), and the lymphomas were listed separately, and the important distinction between cancer of the cervix and other uterine cancers had recently begun. Moreover, by 1950 fairly modern standards of diagnostic radiology already existed, and non-toxic anesthesia and the chemotherapy of infective diseases had just developed, allowing large aseptic operations to help cure abdominal or thoracic cancers that had not already metastasized (and making it less likely that pneumonia or tuberculosis caused by unrecognized primary or secondary cancer in the lung would cause the death of a patient and therefore be miscertified as the underlying cause of death). Finally, although there have been some notable recent advances in the cure of certain leukemias, lymphomas, and tumors of embryomal tissues, there have been no corresponding advances in the cure of the common cancers since 1950 (see appendix C). Therefore, for many cancers the trends since 1950 in death certification rates among people under age 65 are probably a useful indicator of the real trends in disease onset rates in recent decades.

The data for the period since 1950 for the aggregate of all non-respiratory cancers are subdivided (in table D3 for people under 65 and in table D4 for older people) into as much detail as routine Government publications will allow. A more detailed breakdown, covering mortality during 1950–67, is given in the excellent National Cancer Institute Monograph No. 33 (Burbank, 1970); another more detailed breakdown, covering both mortality (1935–74) and incidence (1947–71, comparing the Second and Third National Cancer Surveys, SNCS and TNCS) is given by Devesa and Silverman (1978, 1980). Because Devesa and Silverman did not examine incidence rates separately among people over and under age 65, we have calculated these (table D5).

If attention is restricted to people aged under 65, then for almost all types of cancer except for those strongly affected by smoking (that is, the cancers of the respiratory and upper digestive tracts), the most recent

---

[1] Chiefly lung (and related tissues) but also including the larynx and nasal area but not the pharynx or mouth.

[2] Although the trends in mortality from lung and other respiratory tract cancers do not *of themselves* suggest the existence of any new causes of lung cancer other than cigarettes (and suggest if anything a diminution in the causes other than tobacco of cancer of the larynx and of the aggregate of the remaining respiratory sites apart from the lung), this fact may merely be due to lesser, yet important, effects of other factors being difficult to pick out reliably because of the large effects of cigarettes. For discussion, *see* appendix E.

TABLE D1.—*U.S. age-standardized rates[a] of death certification[b]/100 million people aged under 65 years, 1933–77*

There are at present ≈100 million ♂ and 100 million ♀ under 65 years old in the United States, so the cited rates are roughly similar in magnitude to the actual annual numbers of such deaths.

The 18 age-specific death rates from non-respiratory cancer for 1933–77 and for 1973–77 are compared in text-figures C1 and C2 on page 1272.

Type of cancer	Rates[a]/100 million people, aged under 65 yr, for:									
	Earlier years[b]				More recent years					
	1933–37 (≈1935)	1938–42 (≈1940)	1943–47 (≈1945)	1948–52 (≈1950)	1953–57 (≈1955)	1958–62 (≈1960)	1963–67 (≈1965)	1968–72 (≈1970)	1973–77 (≈1975)	1978 only
Males										
All causes except neoplasms[c]	784,512	675,405	598,171	505,815	448,428	435,853	433,092	423,715	370,013	338,899
All neoplasms except respiratory cancers (*see* text-fig. C1)	58,709	60,226	60,800	59,609	57,938	57,176	57,390	55,282	53,356	52,538
Respiratory cancers	5,812	8,517	11,818	15,498	19,495	23,230	26,766	30,683	32,748	33,816
Females										
All causes except neoplasms[c]	564,675	455,557	372,001	283,429	233,621	219,565	211,012	201,097	171,834	157,607
All neoplasms except respiratory cancers (*see* text-fig. C2)	90,108	87,716	84,401	77,197	71,893	68,765	66,863	63,719	60,574	58,618
Respiratory cancers	2,102	2,450	2,889	2,785	2,820	3,539	4,922	7,568	10,266	12,064

[a] There are moderate uncertainties in the Census Bureau estimates of the age/sex-specific numbers of people at risk of death in each year, especially prior to 1950. (*See* appendix A for standardization methods and appendix B for the population estimates we have used, which differ from those used by other authors.) Also, we are so uncertain as to how well, in the past or in the present, the distinction between "white" and "nonwhite" on death certificates corresponds unbiasedly with that on census returns that only "proportional mortality" analyses of race-specific data seem justifiable. We have therefore presented our analysis of absolute death rates only for all races combined, ignoring estimates of skin color.

[b] There are large uncertainties in the correctness of the *certified* causes of death, especially in the earlier years. Patients dying of cancer of one site might be miscertified as dying of cancer of some other site, or perhaps as dying of a non-cancerous cause (if, for example, the cancer caused or triggered fatal pneumonia, tuberculosis or cerebral disease). For example, in the earlier periods, secondary deposits in the lung from cancers elsewhere were sometimes miscertified as lung cancers; conversely, true primary lung cancers were often not certified as respiratory cancer. Such errors will, of course, be more common among older people, but even among people under 65 years old, the development by the early 1950's of radiology and of aseptic techniques for reasonably safe open-chest and other diagnostic and curative operations would bias the mortality trends in the early years. (It is uncertain whether there has been material progress during the past quarter century in the cure rates among people under 65 years old for the *common* cancers.) People whose age at death was unspecified are ignored in all tables of age-standardized or age-specific mortality.

[c] Benign or malignant, solid or diffuse. Age-specific death rates for Hodgkin's disease, which is nowadays considered to be a neoplasm, were estimated for the period 1939–48 as 91% (the appropriate percentage if the all-ages data for 1939–48 are aggregated) of those for all "other infectious" causes of death.

trends in mortality are downward (last column in table D3) rather than upward. The chief exceptions are pancreatic cancer in women and melanoma in both sexes.

The recent trends (expressed as the percent change per annum in the two separate age-standardized rates both under and over age 65) in the more common cancers are summarized in text-figure D1. There is a general tendency for the rates of change under age 65 to be slightly more favorable than those in old age. The tumor types that stand out most clearly from this general relationship are skin cancer in males (where the increases are much more rapid among people under age 65, unfortunately suggesting that the increases in melanoma will continue for at least the rest of this century and probably beyond) and brain tumors in both sexes (where despite falling death rates in middle age there are large increases in old age, perhaps because of progressive rectification of diagnostic errors; *see* below). Separate discussion of each of the major trends in mortality follows. Because of the methodo-

logical uncertainty (amounting to perhaps ±0.5%/yr) in the incidence trends, we do not discuss them as fully.

Mouth, pharynx, larynx, and esophagus.—These are the sites at which cancers can be caused by alcohol and by tobacco (including pipe tobacco, which men have used since the last century). Few women previously smoked pipes, which may explain why marked upward trends are evident for such cancers only in women. The combination of both alcohol and tobacco exposure seems to cause an increase in the risk of these cancers which greatly exceeds the sum of the two separate risks (*see* section 5.2). The incidence data are distorted by the inclusion in the SNCS but not in the TNCS of salivary gland tumors of "mixed" histology (which are easily cured in most cases).

Other respiratory.—Since 1968, this category has included mesothelioma of the pleura and carcinoma of the nasal sinuses, two types of cancer that can be caused by certain occupational hazards. The absolute risk is low (under 900 males and 500 females in 1978 were certified as dying of "other respiratory" cancers),

TABLE D2.—*U.S. age-standardized rates[a] of death certification[b]/10 million people aged 65 years or over, 1933–77*

There are at present ≈10 million ♂ and 10 million ♀ 65 years old or over in the United States, so the cited rates are roughly similar in magnitude to the actual annual numbers of such deaths.

Because this table relates wholly to people over 65 years old, all the cancer rates in it are likely to be somewhat unreliable, but the rates for the earlier years are even more unreliable than those for the more recent years.[b]

See table D1 for explanations of footnote letters.

Type of cancer	Rates[b]/10 million people, aged 65 yr or over, for:									
	Earlier years[b]				More recent years					
	1933–37 (≈1935)	1938–42 (≈1940)	1943–47 (≈1945)	1948–52 (≈1950)	1953–57 (≈1955)	1958–62 (≈1960)	1963–67 (≈1965)	1968–72 (≈1970)	1973–77 (≈1975)	1978 only
Males										
All causes except neoplasms[c]	815,135	771,843	722,222	682,546	655,477	661,568	657,897	626,788	564,631	528,501
All neoplasms except respiratory cancers (*see* text-fig. C1)	89,921	92,710	92,995	93,837	94,539	91,907	91,708	91,726	94,071	96,436
Respiratory cancers	3,382	4,966	6,899	11,095	15,766	20,471	26,296	33,575	39,511	43,024
Females										
All causes except neoplasms[c]	691,566	640,736	587,619	524,603	486,660	464,038	435,145	398,603	345,983	319,529
All neoplasms except respiratory cancers (*see* text-fig. C2)	84,834	83,139	80,563	76,162	72,575	67,776	65,031	63,745	63,517	64,281
Respiratory cancers	1,473	1,872	2,354	3,050	3,078	3,090	3,551	5,020	6,894	8,672

Footnotes for tables D3, D4, and D6

[a,b,c] *See* footnotes to table D1.

[d] The standard error of a 1978 single-year rate, by the Poisson approximation, is roughly its square root (e.g., a rate of 900 would have a standard error of about ±30).

[e] These are the cancers that are strongly affected both by alcohol and by all forms of tobacco, including the pipes which men smoked in the last century (*see* sections 5.1 and 5.2). The trends in all four cancers are, not surprisingly, rather similar.

[f] Lung (including trachea and bronchus) cancer rates are affected more strongly by cigarette than by pipe smoking (*see* section 5.1), and the increases in respiratory cancer among people under 65 yr old during the past quarter century can be chiefly ascribed to prior widespread adoption of cigarette smoking. (*See* appendix E. There is no *good* evidence of any substantial increases in lung cancer death certification rates among non-smokers under 65 yr old during this period.)

[g] Cancer of the intestines may arise in the small intestine, in the ascending, transverse, descending or sigmoid colon, or in the rectum. U.S. mortality data do not seem to be sufficiently precise to allow unbiased examination of the trends for *any* of the separate parts of the intestines (*see* text), not even for "colon" and "rectum."

[h] Liver, excluding cases where cancer was merely stated to be in the liver, but including cases specified as primary cancer of the liver or of the bile ducts inside the liver.

[i] Gallbladder, including the bile ducts outside the liver.

[j] Mesentery, peritoneum, and unspecified digestive sites (the latter comprising the minority in 1948, when separate totals were last published).

[k] In middle age there are now so few deaths from non-melanoma skin cancers that the data for "total skin" represent the melanoma death rates reasonably accurately, but in old age the continuing decrease in the death rates from non-melanoma skin cancers still dilutes the progressive increase in melanoma death rates [*see* Burbank (1971)].

[l] "Other urinary organs" (ureter and urethra, in which cancers are rare) were included with "bladder" up to 1967, and were then transferred to "kidney" from 1968 onwards.

[m] Endometrium, including all cancers of unspecified parts of the uterus and hence some incompletely described cancers of the uterine cervix, especially in the earlier years.

[n] The distinction between "malignant" and "benign" is less clear-cut for brain tumors than for most other neoplasms, and so the most meaningful analysis seems to be of all fatal tumors of the central nervous system, irrespective of histology. Even here, however, large biases are possible, for in older people, symptoms due to brain tumors may be misdiagnosed as due to senility or vascular disease. Such errors, of course, are less likely for brain tumors that develop in middle age, which may account for the marked upward trend in brain tumor death *certification* rates for the old being entirely absent for people in middle age.

[o] There is considerable diagnostic uncertainty among lymphosarcoma, reticulum cell sarcoma, and various other lymphomas, so we have not attempted to examine them separately. Myeloma was also included because data on myeloma were published separately only from 1968. (Since 1968, the myeloma death *certification* rates for each sex have been increasing at 1.2%/annum among people under 65 years old and at 3.2%/annum among older people.)

[p] On many death certificates, the anatomic site of origin of the cancerous cells that killed the patient is not recorded. This means that for the various specified sites which we have listed separately, the true rates may be a few percent higher than the listed rates. In years when any distinction between "other specified" and "unspecified" sites can be made from U.S. government publications, the unspecified site death certificates greatly outnumber the specified site certificates, although the distinction between them seems surprisingly erratic (e.g., when the rates for 1957 and 1958 are compared).

TABLE D3.—*U.S. age-standardized rates[a] of death certification[b]/100 million people aged under 65 years, 1953–78, from various cancers or groups of cancers[c]*

There are currently ≈100 million people of each sex under 65 years old, so the cited rates are roughly similar in magnitude to the actual annual numbers of such deaths. Consequently, the 1978 single-year rates that are under 1,000 are rather unreliable.[d]

See table D1 and page 1283 for explanation of footnote letters.

Type of cancer	Patients' sex	Rates[b]/100 million people, aged under 65 yr, for:						Current (1968–78) rate of change	
		1953–57 (≈1955)	1958–62 (≈1960)	1963–67 (≈1965)	1968–72 (≈1970)	1973–77 (≈1975)	1978 only	Absolute change/ yr	Percent change/ yr
Mouth, pharynx, larynx, or oesophagus[e]	♂	5,936	6,485	6,858	7,059	7,123	7,200	+8	+0.1
	♀	1,213	1,478	1,700	2,000	2,143	2,111	+25	+1.2
Trachea, bronchus, and lung[f]	♂	—	—	—	28,799	30,911	32,080	+413	+1.4
	♀	—	—	—	7,133	9,803	11,598	+554	+6.3
Other respiratory sites (including pleura and nasal sinus)	♂	—	—	—	475	447	408	−8	−1.8
	♀	—	—	—	215	192	178	−5	−2.6
Sub-total: all respiratory sites except larynx	♂	18,275	21,290	25,390	29,274	31,358	32,488	—	—
	♀	2,714	3,378	4,734	7,348	9,995	11,776	—	—
Stomach	♂	6,808	5,539	4,478	3,753	3,270	2,983	−98	−2.8
	♀	3,293	2,717	2,216	1,815	1,551	1,403	−55	−3.3
Intestines, chiefly large intestine (colon and rectum)[g]	♂	8,954	8,739	8,624	8,521	8,298	8,276	−31	−0.4
	♀	9,014	8,576	7,977	7,486	7,130	6,807	−86	−1.2
Liver[h]	♂	—	—	—	807	795	789	0	0.0
	♀	—	—	—	354	347	383	+2	+0.4
Gallbladder and ducts[i]	♂	—	—	—	535	488	487	−9	−1.7
	♀	—	—	—	712	644	625	−16	−2.4
Sub-total: liver, gallbladder, and bile ducts	♂	1,203	1,396	1,362	1,342	1,283	1,277	—	—
	♀	1,520	1,425	1,219	1,066	991	1,008	—	—
Pancreas	♂	3,984	4,336	4,536	4,464	4,267	4,148	−40	−0.9
	♀	2,210	2,363	2,459	2,482	2,598	2,618	+13	+0.5
Remaining digestive sites, chiefly peritoneum[j]	♂	465	427	404	351	283	256	−13	−4.3
	♀	414	370	330	265	212	193	−10	−4.3
Bone	♂	936	795	747	680	600	575	−14	−2.1
	♀	656	552	483	444	380	360	−11	−2.8
Connective and soft tissue sarcomas	♂	355	419	492	516	464	473	−8	−1.6
	♀	276	338	373	421	414	426	−1	−0.3
Skin, chiefly melanoma[k]	♂	1,325	1,410	1,659	1,547	1,828	1,996	+52	+3.1
	♀	916	935	1,040	1,022	1,086	1,161	+15	+1.4
Breast	♂	138	127	121	130	123	110	−2	−1.2
	♀	15,880	16,158	17,053	17,358	17,260	17,229	−16	−0.1
Bladder[l]	♂	2,066	1,919	1,810	1,658	1,538	1,386	−30	−1.9
	♀	760	676	655	547	500	455	−10	−2.0
Kidney[l]	♂	2,012	2,051	2,134	2,206	2,236	2,300	+6	+0.3
	♀	1,008	1,006	991	1,018	1,016	1,011	0	0.0
Cervix uteri	♀	7,550	6,651	5,673	4,423	3,365	2,911	−206	−5.4
Endometrium[m]	♀	4,218	3,282	2,650	2,193	1,966	1,815	−46	−2.2
Ovary	♀	5,692	5,736	5,680	5,621	5,304	5,042	−68	−1.2
Prostate	♂	2,785	2,602	2,549	2,555	2,612	2,590	+7	+0.3
Other genital sites									
Malignant	♂	854	852	837	811	729	540	−23	−3.0
	♀	356	326	291	274	246	224	−6	−2.4
Possibly benign	♀	835	444	302	173	95	53	−16	−12.2
Brain or nerves, malignant or benign[n]	♂	4,908	4,822	4,831	4,693	4,475	4,293	−47	−1.0
	♀	3,675	3,663	3,653	3,520	3,364	3,246	−35	−1.0
Eye	♂	127	120	102	92	77	70	−3	−3.4
	♀	116	106	100	82	66	58	−3	−4.2
Thyroid	♂	236	207	186	182	153	146	−5	−3.2
	♀	340	304	255	210	177	181	−6	−3.0
Leukemia	♂	4,754	4,843	4,705	4,344	4,036	3,845	−64	−1.5
	♀	3,562	3,477	3,338	3,049	2,753	2,622	−59	−2.0
Hodgkin's disease	♂	1,775	1,770	1,770	1,573	1,065	830	−95	−7.4
	♀	992	999	1,025	918	620	486	−54	−7.2
All other lymphomas[o]	♂	3,603	3,862	4,070	4,429	4,254	4,267	−24	−0.6
	♀	2,260	2,543	2,720	2,884	2,875	2,876	+1	0.0
Other specified and unspecified[p] sites	♂	5,935	5,775	6,490	5,805	6,029	6,304	+57	+1.0
	♀	5,244	4,800	4,868	4,669	4,734	4,613	−2	−0.1

TABLE D4.—*U.S. age-standardized rates[a] of death certification[b]/10 million people aged 65 years or over, 1953–78, from various cancers or groups of cancers[c]*

There are currently ≈10 million Americans of each sex aged 65 years or over, so the cited values are roughly similar in magnitude to the annual numbers of such deaths. Consequently, those 1978 single-year rates that are under 1,000 are rather unreliable.[d]
See table D1 and page 1283 for explanation of footnote letters.

Type of cancer	Patients' sex	Rates[b]/10 million people, aged 65 or over, for:						Current (1968–78) rate of change	
		1953–57 (≈1955)	1958–62 (≈1960)	1963–67 (≈1965)	1968–72 (≈1970)	1973–77 (≈1975)	1978 only	Absolute change/ yr	Percent change/ yr
Mouth, pharynx, larynx, or esophagus[e]	♂	8,027	7,580	7,214	7,324	7,478	7,487	+24	+0.3
	♀	1,786	1,654	1,551	1,643	1,787	1,933	+30	+1.7
Trachea, bronchus, and lung[f]	♂	—	—	—	31,539	37,424	40,888	+1197	+3.4
	♀	—	—	—	4,692	6,550	8,296	+403	+6.9
Other respiratory sites (including pleura and nasal sinus)	♂	—	—	—	483	492	468	+2	+0.3
	♀	—	—	—	205	195	203	−1	−0.7
Sub-total: all respiratory sites except larynx	♂	14,277	19,016	24,823	32,022	37,916	41,356	—	—
	♀	2,937	2,981	3,442	4,897	6,745	8,499	—	—
Stomach	♂	14,368	11,827	9,552	7,708	6,519	5,892	−241	−3.4
	♀	7,547	5,930	4,635	3,667	3,047	2,870	−117	−3.5
Intestines, chiefly large intestine (colon and rectum)[g]	♂	17,916	17,749	17,761	17,958	18,265	18,839	+83	+0.5
	♀	15,502	14,672	14,024	13,497	13,250	10,437	−35	−0.3
Liver[h]	♂	—	—	—	926	957	1,067	+13	+1.3
	♀	—	—	—	364	376	395	+4	+1.0
Gallbladder and ducts[i]	♂	—	—	—	1,267	1,193	1,192	−14	−1.1
	♀	—	—	—	1,749	1,479	1,459	−48	−3.0
Sub-total: liver, gallbladder, and bile ducts	♂	1,921	2,106	2,208	2,193	2,150	2,259	—	—
	♀	2,651	2,561	2,357	2,113	1,855	1,854	—	—
Pancreas	♂	5,816	6,426	6,899	7,090	7,169	7,247	+9	+0.1
	♀	3,842	4,074	4,226	4,390	4,463	4,637	+24	+0.5
Remaining digestive sites, chiefly peritoneum[j]	♂	729	668	628	500	483	417	−7	−1.4
	♀	649	610	540	431	365	317	−13	−3.4
Bone	♂	837	617	521	502	465	436	−8	−1.7
	♀	468	359	308	286	261	244	−6	0.0
Connective and soft tissue sarcomas	♂	228	273	323	357	353	355	+0.4	+0.1
	♀	156	184	209	243	244	273	+3	+1.1
Skin, chiefly melanoma[k]	♂	1,867	1,739	1,679	1,448	1,527	1,608	+15	+1.0
	♀	1,118	961	863	780	789	840	+7	+0.9
Breast	♂	201	166	175	192	188	181	−1	−0.4
	♀	11,356	10,633	10,351	10,603	11,087	11,070	+76	+0.7
Bladder[l]	♂	5,416	5,496	5,501	5,626	5,781	5,732	+23	+0.4
	♀	2,258	2,042	1,876	1,673	1,615	1,623	−10	−0.6
Kidney[l]	♂	1,735	1,969	2,166	2,488	2,543	2,670	+23	+0.9
	♀	1,047	1,066	1,105	1,160	1,222	1,252	+11	+0.9
Cervix uteri	♀	3,127	2,884	2,513	2,021	1,642	1,403	−73	−4.1
Endometrium[m]	♀	4,068	3,512	3,175	2,861	2,662	2,593	−38	−1.4
Ovary	♀	3,195	3,344	3,460	3,680	3,743	3,796	+20	+0.5
Prostate	♂	19,300	18,584	18,488	18,591	19,465	20,392	+183	+1.0
Other genital sites									
Malignant	♂	435	359	320	295	252	224	−9	−3.3
	♀	645	604	545	514	495	470	−5	−1.0
Possibly benign	♀	240	147	115	72	51	39	−5	−7.7
Brain or nerves, malignant or benign[n]	♂	935	1,068	1,375	1,731	2,163	2,581	+98	+4.9
	♀	596	692	857	1,187	1,522	1,862	+75	+5.4
Eye	♂	131	123	106	112	99	102	−1	−1.2
	♀	106	91	79	79	70	64	−3	−2.5
Thyroid	♂	276	251	234	232	210	217	−1	−0.6
	♀	524	450	417	372	338	310	−6	−1.7
Leukemia	♂	3,924	4,512	4,855	5,015	5,053	5,142	+12	+0.2
	♀	2,273	2,474	2,612	2,704	2,609	2,627	−12	−0.4
Hodgkin's disease	♂	626	600	626	592	468	384	−24	−4.6
	♀	388	374	397	385	296	261	−16	−4.9
All other lymphomas[o]	♂	2,701	3,303	3,900	5,126	5,787	6,266	+133	+2.4
	♀	1,849	2,227	2,634	3,470	3,894	4,184	+90	+2.4
Other specified and unspecified[p] sites	♂	8,637	7,945	8,650	8,198	9,248	9,666	+194	+2.2
	♀	7,324	6,341	6,294	6,038	6,354	6,502	+62	+1.0

TABLE D5.—*U.S. age-standardized rates of cancer registration/100 million people under 65 years, 1947–71, from the SNCS, 1947/48, and the TNCS, 1969–71*[a,b]

The trends among "whites only" and the trends among "all races" are both presented (because there has been dispute as to which should be more reliable), although the trends suggested by both are virtually identical.

Type of cancer	Patients' sex	Whites only, aged <65 yr		All races, aged <65 yr		Long-term (1947–70) rate of change, all races	
		SNCS, 1947/48	TNCS, 1969–71	SNCS, 1947/48	TNCS, 1969–71	Absolute change/ yr[c]	Percent change/ yr[d]
Mouth, esophagus, pharynx, and larynx	♂	21,355	17,795	21,154	18,710	−109	−0.5
	♀	5,389	5,309	5,628	5,609	−1	−0.01
Trachea, bronchus, lung, and other respiratory sites except larynx	♂	22,022	37,435	21,966	39,038	+759	+2.6
	♀	4,996	10,223	5,070	10,209	+228	+3.1
Stomach	♂	16,083	4,795	17,303	5,290	−534	−5.3
	♀	7,757	2,279	8,277	2,446	−259	−5.4
Intestines, chiefly colon and rectum	♂	25,446	20,261	24,446	20,353	−182	−0.8
	♀	24,871	17,092	24,434	17,195	−322	−1.6
Liver[e]	♂	2,969	1,321	3,120	1,613	−67	−2.9
	♀	2,046	653	2,099	666	−64	−5.1
Gallbladder and bile ducts	♂	1,100	967	1,097	966	−6	−0.6
	♀	2,485	991	2,376	1,015	−60	−3.8
Pancreas	♂	4,737	4,828	4,770	5,100	+15	+0.3
	♀	2,976	2,761	3,066	2,933	−6	−0.2
Remaining digestive sites	♂	1,375	981	1,328	1,001	−15	−1.3
	♀	1,174	953	1,146	944	−9	−0.9
Bones[e]	♂	1,959	805	2,029	822	−54	−4.0
	♀	1,687	596	1,583	579	−45	−4.5
Connective and soft tissue	♂	1,545	1,505	1,708	1,550	−7	−0.4
	♀	1,581	1,346	1,520	1,385	−6	−0.4
Skin[f]		—	—	—	—	—	—
Breast	♂	436	349	413	344	−3	−0.8
	♀	52,343	54,132	50,982	53,367	+106	+0.2
Bladder only	♂	8,626	8,784	8,134	8,448	+14	+0.2
	♀	3,410	2,507	3,667	2,399	−56	−1.9
Kidney only	♂	3,906	4,716	3,837	4,747	+40	+0.9
	♀	1,955	2,367	1,879	2,379	+22	+1.0
Cervix uteri	♀	27,751	12,740	31,231	14,245	−755	−3.5
Endometrium and uterus, site unspecified	♀	17,712	16,974	17,614	16,336	−57	−0.3
Ovary	♀	12,361	10,365	11,984	10,105	−83	−0.8
Prostate	♂	7,178	10,249	8,182	11,275	+137	+1.4
Other genital sites	♂	2,770	4,026	2,774	3,787	+45	+1.4
	♀	2,139	1,596	2,167	1,728	−20	−1.0
Brain[g]	♂	6,820	4,950	6,487	4,767	−76[g]	−1.4[g]
	♀	4,885	3,710	4,766	3,663	−49[g]	−1.2[g]
Eye[h]		—	—	—	—	—	—
Thyroid	♂	957	1,818	838	1,716	+39	+3.2
	♀	2,799	4,725	2,720	4,532	+81	+2.3
Leukemia	♂	6,206	6,315	6,143	6,181	+2	+0.03
	♀	5,156	4,001	4,791	3,952	−37	−0.9
Hodgkin's disease	♂	2,976	3,549	2,907	3,440	+24	+0.7
	♀	2,267	2,302	2,149	2,145	0	0.0
All other lymphomas	♂	5,350	6,475	5,429	6,575	+51	+0.9
	♀	3,726	4,249	3,774	4,414	+28	+0.7
Other specified and unspecified[i] sites, including eye[h]	♂	8,618	6,335	8,687	6,636	−91	−1.2
	♀	9,394	4,675	9,326	4,874	−198	−2.9
Sub-total, all respiratory sites, including larynx	♂	26,910	42,501	26,712	44,167	+776	+2.2
	♀	5,430	10,968	5,511	10,976	+243	+3.1
Sub-total, non-respiratory and unspecified sites, excluding skin	♂	125,524	105,757	126,037	108,173	−794	−0.7
	♀	195,431	155,576	196,738	156,144	−1804	−1.0

[a] Data and population estimates from PHS monograph 29 (1955) and NCI monograph 41 (1975).

[b] For details of age standardization procedure, *see* appendix A.

[c] Estimated as difference in rates divided by 22.5 yr.

[d] Estimated as 100% × difference in log$_e$ rate(s) divided by 22.5 yr.

[e] The downward trends in liver and bone cancer registration rates may be largely attributable to a progressive reduction in misdiagnosis, because these are sites to which other types of cancer commonly metastasize. (*Note* that in the TNCS, but not in the SNCS, "joints" were explicitly included with "bones.")

[f] SNCS included all skin cancers while TNCS included only melanomas, so trends in skin cancer incidence cannot be estimated from a comparison of these two surveys.

[g] Non-malignant brain tumors were counted in the Second but not in the Third Survey, so the apparent decrease in brain tumors is uninformative.

[h] Tumors of the eye were not listed separately in SNCS.

[i] The decrease in this category is chiefly due to a decrease in the number of tumors of an unspecified site. This artifactual decrease (and the similar decreases in secondary tumors mis-specified as liver or bone) must imply corresponding artifactual increases (of the order of 0.1%/yr) in many of the specified sites.

TABLE D6.—*U.S. death certification rates/10 million people aged 35–44 years,[q] 1968–78, from various cancers or groups of cancers[a,b,c,d]*
There are currently ≈10 million Americans of each sex aged 35–44 years.
See table D1 and page 1283 for explanation of footnote letters.

Type of cancer	Patients' sex	Rates/10 million Americans, all races, aged 35–44 yr[q]			
		1968–72 (≈1970)	1973–77 (≈1975)	1978 rate ± SE[r]	Change, 1970–78, and significance level[s]
Mouth, pharynx, larynx or esophagus[e]	♂	296	281	271±15	−25
	♀	114	103	95±9	−19*
Trachea, bronchus, and lung[f]	♂	1,446	1,347	1,232±32	−214***
	♀	601	676	698±24	+97***
Other respiratory sites	♂	38	34	35±5	−3
	♀	21	15	17±4	−4
Stomach	♂	200	188	159±11	−41**
	♀	160	122	123±10	−37**
Intestines, chiefly colon and rectum[g]	♂	437	422	426±19	−11
	♀	473	433	377±18	−96***
Liver[h,i]	♂	43	42	50±6	+7[t]
	♀	31	27	31±5	0
Gallbladder and ducts[i]	♂	27	21	21±4	−6
	♀	30	30	26±5	−4
Pancreas	♂	224	196	167±12	−57***
	♀	128	122	109±9	−19*
Remaining digestive sites, chiefly peritoneum[j]	♂	24	19	18±4	−6
	♀	23	14	20±4	−3
Bone	♂	34	35	32±5	−2
	♀	29	21	19±4	−10*
Connective and soft tissue sarcomas	♂	49	49	48±6	−1
	♀	42	39	38±6	−4
Skin, chiefly melanoma[k]	♂	222	240	284±15	+62***
	♀	175	172	169±12	−6
Breast	♂	9	9	8±3	−1
	♀	1,969	1,807	1,716±37	−253***
Bladder[l]	♂	42	35	25±5	17**
	♀	22	20	12±3	−10**
Kidney[l]	♂	128	129	130±10	+2
	♀	68	61	60±7	−8
Cervix uteri	♀	717	530	461±19	−256***
Endometrium[m]	♀	146	109	110±10	−36***
Ovary	♀	481	400	328±16	−153***
Prostate	♂	16	15	10±3	−6*
Other genital sites					
Malignant	♂	115	98	80±8	−35***
	♀	23	19	12±3	−11**
Possibly benign	♀	42	21	12±3	−30***
Brain or nerves, malignant or benign[n]	♂	440	412	387±18	−53**
	♀	346	311	280±15	−66***
Eye	♂	5	5	3±2	−2
	♀	5	4	2±1	−3
Thyroid	♂	14	11	12±3	−2
	♀	15	12	9±3	−6*
Leukemia	♂	324	292	299±16	−25
	♀	267	245	251±14	−16
Hodgkin's disease	♂	226	154	125±10	−101***
	♀	125	83	68±7	−57***
All other lymphomas[o]	♂	329	286	305±16	−24
	♀	207	190	177±12	−30*
Other specified and unspecified[p] sites	♂	367	348	328±16	−39*
	♀	379	356	350±17	−29
Total, all sites, all histologies	♂	5,054	4,670	4,454±60	−600***
	♀	6,638	5,942	5,571±68	−1,067***

[q] Rates estimated as average of rates at 35–39 and at ages 40–44 yr.
[r] SE denotes the standard error of the 1978 rate. The standard errors of the other two rates (1968–72 and 1973–77) are both ≈0.5 SE, while the standard error of the change (1968–72 to 1978) is ≈1.1 SE.
[s] *, **, *** denote $P<0.1$, $P<0.01$, $P<0.001$, respectively (two-tailed test). The change was estimated by subtraction of the 1978 rate from the 1968–72 rate.
[t] The increase in liver cancer death among males aged 35–44 yr in 1978 would be of interest if real, but it is not statistically significant (62 deaths observed in 1978 vs. 52.3 expected on the basis of the 1968–77 death rates), and corresponding increases are not seen among males aged 15–34 yr nor among males aged 45–64 yr. The slightly high rate among men aged 35–44 yr in 1978 is, therefore, probably largely or wholly an artifact of chance.

TEXT-FIGURE D1.—Trends in U.S. cancer death certification rates for cancers that are common in middle or old age: Relationship between trends above and below age 65 years.

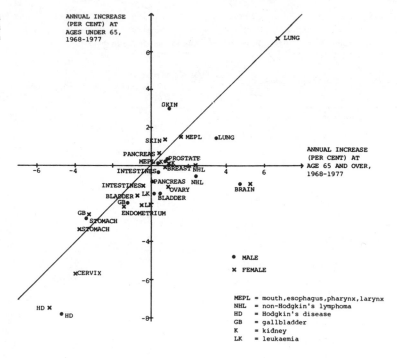

and it is striking that it shows no upward trend. This may be partly because the trends in pleural and nasal sinus cancers are opposite in direction and cancel each other out (Burbank, 1970) and partly because of a progressive tendency for doctors to avoid such imprecise terms as cancer of the "mediastinum" or "thoracic organs" in death certification. (In Britain, where a more detailed subdivision of these "other respiratory" cancers is published, the percentage of the small number of male "other respiratory" cancers that were pleural increased from 36% in 1968–72 to 56% in 1978, whereas the percentage that were mediastinal decreased from 12 to 5%.)

Stomach.—Stomach cancer is now decreasing throughout the developed world (table 5 on page 1202), even though the case fatality rate is still about 90%. None of the dietary explanations involving reductions in contamination by micro-organisms of food due to modern food processing or storage have been either accepted or rejected, possibly because it is the diet during childhood or early adult life that largely determines the risk in middle or old age, an association that would be difficult to study epidemiologically. The enormously encouraging feature of the U.S. stomach cancer trends is that they are continuing downward in each age group *throughout middle age,* which strongly suggests that the decreases occurring in old age will continue throughout this century and perhaps beyond. The United States, which used to have very high stomach cancer rates, already has incidence rates that are among the lowest recorded in any country in the world, and

hopefully the decreases in the United States will be a model that other countries will continue to follow.

Intestines.—On death certificates, intestinal cancer may be of either a specified or an unspecified part of the intestines. In 1958, about two-thirds of male intestinal cancer deaths were certified as being of some *specified*[3] intestinal site, and one-third were of an *unspecified* intestinal site, whereas by 1977 the converse was true. Overall, little change occurred in total male intestinal cancer mortality during this period. Clearly, although the male death certification rates for each specific intestinal site have been approximately halved, these decreases cannot be accepted as real because the unspecified site rates have doubled. However, it has been traditional to present the data for one particular specific site ("rectum," comprising the last foot or so of the large intestine) separately and to describe the remainder, including unspecified intestinal sites, as "colon." This approach gives the misleading impression that rectal cancer rates are really decreasing and colon cancer rates are really increasing, whereas in fact the decreases in the death certification rates for rectum are, if anything, slightly less extreme than for many of the other (colonic) specified parts of the intestines. In view of the fact that half of all fatal cancers diagnosed in hospital as "rectum" in the TNCS were eventually

---

[3] Small intestine, ascending colon, transverse colon, descending colon, sigmoid colon, or rectum.

certified as "colon," the most plausible interpretation of the data is that there have been no material trends in either colon or rectal cancer mortality during the past quarter of a century among males, though both the mortality and some incidence data do suggest a slight decrease in onset rates below age 65. Similar difficulties of classification affect females, and when all intestinal sites are combined total female intestinal cancer death rates have been decreasing steadily since 1950.

Liver.—The human liver is a large organ, intimately exposed to much of what is ingested and composed of cells that are capable of rapid proliferation when necessary. Moreover, most of the chemicals that have thus far been found to be carcinogenic in animal feeding experiments cause liver cancer in animals (and one in particular, aflatoxin B_1, seems capable of doing likewise in humans). It is therefore of interest to note that among Americans under age 65 liver cancer currently accounts for only 0.8% of cancer death certificates, and that no statistically significant trends in liver cancer mortality are evident during the past decade. (Human liver cancer is still rapidly fatal in almost all cases, so neither the absolute mortality rates nor the trends can have been materially affected by improvements in therapy.) The decreases in incidence (table D5) are presumably chiefly artifactual due to the improving differential diagnosis between primary and secondary liver cancer.

Gallbladder and bile ducts.—Cancers of these two sites have different causes, gallstones being an important risk factor for the gallbladder. The two sites are unfortunately not reported separately either in mortality data or in the published incidence data from the SNCS in 1947/48. They are, however, reported separately in the TNCS (1969-71), in which the sex ratios are opposite, females developing cancer of the gallbladder rather than of the bile ducts.[4]

Tables D3, D4, and D5 indicate that decreases have occurred and are continuing to occur in the aggregate of these two types of cancers and that these decreases are larger among females than among males. This finding suggests that it is probably cancer of the gallbladder that is chiefly decreasing, rather than cancer of the bile ducts. However, since, like liver cancer, both diseases are commonly fatal (with 5-yr relative survival rates <10%), the real trends in incidence and mortality must be similar. As this is not what the available data indicate, the true size of the trends remains unknown. If reliable site-specific data were available, the relative decrease in cancer of the gallbladder might be as striking as that in cancer of the stomach. We do not know whether whatever decrease does exist is partly due to a decrease of the biologic causes of the disease or whether it is due simply to

progressively more surgical treatment of gallstones and to removal of more and more of those few gallbladders at greatest risk of gallstone formation.

Pancreas.—It is encouraging that, after increasing for decades, the trend in male pancreatic cancer at ages under 65 is now downward, the decreases in early middle age being particularly rapid. Pancreatic cancer is again so uniformly fatal that treatment cannot have affected these trends. If the correlation of smoking with pancreatic cancer represents a cause-and-effect relationship, one might expect the ratio of rates among smokers and non-smokers to be increasing, as has been true in recent years for lung cancer. If this ratio is indeed increasing, then among middle-aged male non-smokers the trend in pancreatic cancer mortality must be even more steeply downward than these national data suggest (as might the female non-smoker rates). This prediction, and a similar prediction of steeper-than-average downward bladder cancer trends among non-smokers, could easily be checked in the data from the two large prospective studies of U.S. non-smokers.

Remaining digestive.—The decreases in this may be chiefly artifactual, due to transfer of some cancers of an unspecified digestive site either to a wholly unspecified site or to some specified site. Since 1968 "remaining digestive" has included peritoneal mesothelioma, a type of tumor that can be caused by asbestos, but these are so rare (only a few dozen per year in each sex out of a few hundred per year "remaining digestive" in each sex. Cutler and Young, 1975) that their trends cannot be estimated from the trends in "remaining digestive."

Bone.—The apparent decreases in "bone" cancer death certification rates (and incidence rates) may be due chiefly to the progressive elimination of misdiagnosed secondaries (Boyd et al., 1969), though the similar magnitudes of the trends in young and old does not support this.

Skin.—The upward trends in skin cancer mortality during 1950–67 were the sum of an increasing death rate from melanomas, together with a decreasing death rate from other skin tumors (Burbank, 1970). The increases are most rapid in middle age, and so the rates in old age will probably increase even more rapidly in future decades than is already the case. The causes of melanoma are not well understood; exposure to sunlight seems to be involved, and patients with xeroderma pigmentosum, which involves a genetic deficiency in their ability to repair the damage done to their DNA by sunlight, are at extraordinarily high risk of melanoma (Robbins et al., 1974). However, people whose work involves regular outdoor exposure seem paradoxically to be at lower risk of melanoma than otherwise similar people who work indoors (Lee and Strickland, 1980), perhaps because a permanent suntan is protective. Therefore, the conditions that maximize risk may be those that involve sudden exposure of untanned skin to sunlight. It is possible that the worldwide increases in melanoma are due merely to some change in the pattern of human exposure to sunlight (e.g., changes in clothing or increases in

---

[4] At ages <65 in 1969-71, the all-races age-standardized incidence rates per 100 million for cancer of the gallbladder were 573 for females and 305 for males, whereas for cancer of the extrahepatic bile ducts they were 442 for females and 661 for males.

sunbathing), particularly since the chief increases seem to be in melanoma of the trunk and legs rather than of the face (Magnus, 1980). However, melanocytes are also subject to hormonal influences, and it could yet be that other, undiscovered, causes are also important.

Breast.—The lack of any substantial trends in breast cancer incidence or mortality at ages under 65 is deceptive and conceals various smaller fluctuations in mortality in particular age groups, with women born in different decades having differing risks in later life. Delay of first pregnancy is known to be a determinant of breast cancer risk in later life (MacMahon et al., 1973), and Blot (1980) has argued that the reproductive patterns of different cohorts of American women can account for some or all of the small fluctuations in breast cancer death rates in particular cohorts of women. (Women who were young during the Great Depression of the 1930's had their children at a somewhat delayed time, and their breast cancer mortality nowadays is slightly increased, while women who were young in the postwar baby boom now have, in early middle age, substantially decreased breast cancer rates because of their early pregnancies.)

Bladder.—The steady decrease in bladder cancer death rates in both sexes is encouraging, since bladder cancer can be caused by occupational exposure to various carcinogens. [Blot and Fraumeni (1975) report similar decreases in the industrial Northeast of the United States, despite a heavy concentration of chemical manufacturing industries there.] However, the discrepancy between rising incidence and falling mortality is more marked for bladder than for any other type of cancer except thyroid cancer (*see* below). This divergence may be contributed to by improvements in treatment, but the reason why it is peculiarly extreme is probably because there is no sharp distinction between bladder "papillomas" and bladder "carcinomas," and by now a substantial proportion of the bladder "cancers" counted by certain registries are what clinicians or histologists in the past might have classified as "papillomas" (Muir, 1976).

Kidney.—At ages under 65, small increases in male (but, until recently, not female) kidney cancer death certification rates have been continuing for 25 years, together with slightly larger increases in incidence in both sexes. Men who smoke cigarettes have mutagenic urine (Yamasaki and Ames, 1977), a marked excess of bladder cancer (*see* section 5.1), and about a 40% excess of kidney cancer in both of the large American prospective studies. It is not known whether this excess is an artifact of the epidemiologic method, but if not then it could account for the small upward trend in mortality from cancer of the kidney.

Cervix, endometrium, and ovary.—Large decreases in mortality from cancer of the uterine cervix have continued throughout the past half century at least, were apparent long before screening for cancer of the cervix became widespread, and are the chief reason for the large, steady decrease in female non-respiratory death rates over the past 40 years. The causes of this

substantial improvement are not fully understood, though effects of improved personal hygiene may be relevant. It is not known what the current trends in cervix cancer mortality would be were it not for the benefits of cervical cancer screening programs. Also, if all of the deaths between 1933 and 1978 from cancer of the cervix that were certified merely as being due to "cancer of the uterus" (with the exact site not otherwise specified) could be transferred from "endometrium," where they now are, to "cervix," the downward trend in cancer of the cervix would presumably be much steeper and that from cancer of the endometrium much shallower. This suggestion is supported by the trends in recorded incidence in table D5. Finally, an increasing percentage of American women in middle and old age, when cancer is most common, have already undergone hysterectomy for various reasons, thereby removing both cervix uteri and endometrium (and, sometimes, both ovaries) from risk. A better statistic might be the death rate from such cancers per uterus, not per woman (and, likewise, in ovarian cancer per ovary), and the recent trends in these rates would presumably seem somewhat less encouraging. They might well indicate no material decrease in cancer of the endometrium, though the decreases in cancer of the cervix seem far too large to be accounted for by any combination of the above sources of error.

Brain.—The distinction between malignant brain tumors, benign brain tumors, and brain tumors of unspecified malignancy is not reliable, and so all three must be pooled if meaningful analyses, especially of trends, are to emerge. Because of the possibility of diagnostic confusion between brain tumors and other brain diseases in old people, separate examination of the death rates among people under age 65 and those among older people is perhaps more important for brain tumors than for any other category of neoplasm (text-fig. D1). Under age 65, we see a 1% per annum decrease in brain tumor death certification rates. Over age 65 the opposite is true, and a very rapid increase in death certification rates exists, possibly due to a steady improvement of diagnostic standards. Future death certification and, particularly, registered incidence rates may be further increased as the diagnostic accuracy conferred by computerized transaxial tomograms ("EMI-scans") and other special investigations becomes more and more widely available.

Thyroid.—The contrast between steadily falling death certification rates and the outstandingly rapid increase in incidence suggested by table D5 is greater for thyroid cancer than for any other type of tumor and may in part be explained by the epidemic of non-fatal thyroid cancers induced by medical use of X-rays.

Hodgkin's disease and certain forms of leukemia.— These diseases are much more treatable now than they were a decade or two ago. This alone will produce substantial downward trends in mortality, especially among younger people (*see* table C2), and may perhaps have encouraged more thorough efforts at correct diagnosis, especially among older people. Reliable estimation of separate trends in the various different types of leukemia is, unfortunately, not possible from the available data due to lack of consistent classification and terminology. The lack of any net trend in either direction in leukemia mortality among older people may represent a balance between increasingly thorough diagnosis among elderly patients who are dying of leukemia and slightly better treatment of the disease. It is not possible in this situation to know whether the underlying age-specific leukemia onset rates are changing, but the incidence data do suggest that some decreases in real onset rates are in progress, at least among females.

All other tumors of the reticuloendothelial system.— These tumors comprise several different diseases, none of which (except possibly myeloma) can be studied separately, again because of a lack of consistent diagnostic criteria. Among people under age 65, for whom no net trends in mortality are evident, rising incidence may be balanced by better treatment; or perhaps no material trends exist in lymphoma onset rates, but (as for leukemia) better case ascertainment is being balanced by better treatment.

Death certification rates from myelomatosis have been rising steadily during 1968-78 (1.2±0.3%/year among people under age 65 and 3.2±0.2%/year among older people). This difference between the rates of increase in middle and in old age might be the tail end of the sort of "successive generation effect" described for smoking and lung cancer in appendix E. Alternatively, it might simply mean that the apparent increase in myelomatosis is largely or wholly due merely to improved case finding rather than to increased incidence, because improved case finding must have occurred during 1968-78 and might be expected to have its greatest effect among the old. (Recent improvements in diagnostic technology could cause particularly large upward biases in myeloma death certification rates, because the disease may present acutely as terminal renal failure or bone marrow failure, and the correct diagnosis could easily be missed if electrophoretic blood protein analyses are not undertaken.)

Other and unspecified sites.—Of all cancers at ages under 65, 6-8% are of an unspecified site, the exact percentage varying irregularly since 1950, with, rather surprisingly, slight increases during the past decade.

"Early" and "Late"-Acting Determinants of Cancer: The Crucial Importance of Trends in Cancer in Early Middle Age

The different trends in the death certification rates for each separate type of cancer have a variety of different causes, and each must therefore be discussed separately. Some general points can, however, be made about the surprisingly long delays that typically seem to exist between cause and effect in carcinogenesis. For many types of cancer the cancerous alteration of a normal cell is thought to involve the accumulation, over several decades, of at least two different sorts of

permanent, or semi-permanent, change in particular cells, such that it is only a cell that has suffered the "early" change(s) that is at risk of the "late" change(s) that will finally convert it into the seed of a growing cancer. (For review, *see* Peto, 1977.) If this theory, or anything roughly equivalent to it, is true, then the determinants of cancer can perhaps be divided into three main classes: *a)* those that principally affect only the "early" stages, *b)* those that principally affect only the "late" stages, and *c)* those that have a substantial effect on both early and late stages. Theoretically, tripling the likelihood of the early stages occurring triples the risk of cancer, as does tripling (among cells that have already undergone their "early" changes) the likelihood of the late stages occurring, whereas doing both might increase the final risk of cancer ninefold.

Again, whether or not this is exactly true, the risk of cancer in old age is strongly dependent both on the rate of occurrence of the "early" changes in one's cells during childhood or early adult life, and on the rate of occurrence, among cells that have undergone the early change(s), of the "late" change(s) in middle or old age. Clearly, if the early changes are increased or decreased then it may be 50 years or more before the full effects of this on national mortality data are evident, whereas if the later stages are increased (e.g., by post-menopausal hormones) or decreased (e.g., by stopping smoking, since smoking seems to affect both the early and the late stages of lung carcinogenesis—*see* appendix E) then measurable effects may be seen within a decade.

If there were no general upward trend in current cancer onset rates, this would suggest that recent changes in the American life-style or environment have not grossly affected the "later" processes of induction of most cancers, but it would not offer any guarantee against significant increases or decreases during the past quarter of a century in the rates of occurrence of the "early" stages. However, separate examination of the trends in mortality among adults in *early* middle age might reveal more clearly any adverse or beneficial tendencies in exposure to early-stage carcinogens. We have therefore tabulated separately the trends in cancer death rates observed during the 1970's among Americans aged 35-44 (table D6). The absolute numbers of deaths involved are very small, which introduces difficulties of statistical significance that did not affect the earlier tables. However, where statistically significant trends in one or another direction can be demonstrated among people currently aged 35-44, the directions of these significant trends are of crucial importance, because they offer some of the best clues there are as to the likely direction of the trends in cancer mortality that will be seen in the 1980's among people aged 45-54, in the 1990's among people aged 55-64, and among old people early in the next century.

The significant patterns in table D6 seem to be:
a) Continuation at ages 35-44 of the *upward* trends already noted above among older people in cancer of the lung (females only) and skin (males only).
b) Continuation at ages 35-44 of the *downward*

trends already noted above among older people in cancer of the stomach (both sexes), intestines (females only), ovary, endometrium, cervix uteri and other parts of the female reproductive system, brain (both sexes), bladder (both sexes), and in Hodgkin's disease (both sexes). The decrease in Hodgkin's disease is largely or wholly ascribable to effective treatment, but this seems unlikely to be true on the whole of these other significant decreases.

c) Recent emergence of very marked decreases in mortality at ages 35–44 from cancer of the male lung, female breast, and pancreas (chiefly in men, but perhaps also in women). At least two of these three trends are very encouraging. The decrease in male lung cancer is encouraging because it suggests that a peak in the still-evolving epidemic of male lung cancer can now be foreseen. (See text-fig. E3 on page 0000 for more detail; in appendix E the decrease in lung cancer mortality among younger men is attributed more to decreasing tar yields than to decreasing cigarette consumption.) The decrease in male (and perhaps female) pancreatic cancer might also be at least in part due to decreases in exposure to the affects of tobacco (see section 5.1) if smoking effects chiefly the later stages of pancreatic cancer induction. Pancreatic cancer remains almost wholly incurable, yet peak rates for cancer of the pancreas among middle-aged males were reached in the mid-1960's. Since then, decreases have occurred throughout middle age, but most especially in early middle age for which unexplained decreases of about 30% have already been recorded. The marked decrease in mortality at ages 35–44 from cancer of the female breast is perhaps less encouraging, for it may merely indicate a protective effect of early pregnancy only on the mothers of the postwar baby boom (Blot, 1980), in which case the decreases seen in table D6 will presumably be replaced in a decade or two by increases in breast cancer in early middle age due to the delayed fertility of the 1960's and 1970's.

When one considers the aggregate of all types of cancer at ages 35–44, male death rates decreased by 12% between 1970 and 1978, whereas female rates decreased by 16%. These decreases are produced by the sum of many factors, but even if the effects of any "one-off" improvements in cancer therapy (and any temporary effects of the postwar baby boom) are allowed for, the net trends would still seem favorable. It is therefore reasonable to hope that the overall decreases seen during the 1970's in cancer death rates among Americans aged 35–44 will be seen at older ages around the turn of the century. The trends in lung cancer are discussed more fully in appendix E.

APPENDIX E: TRENDS IN LUNG CANCER DEATH RATES IN RELATION TO CIGARETTE USAGE AND TAR YIELDS

Effects of Smoking in Early and Recent Adult Life

As would be expected, lung cancer risks at 60 years of age depend strongly on the degree of exposure of the lungs to cigarette smoke over the previous decade or so. The chief evidence for this assertion is that a) people aged 60 who have given up smoking 10 years previously have lung cancer risks that are well under half the risks among continuing cigarette smokers (Rogot and Murray, 1980; Doll and Peto, 1976; Hammond, 1966) and that b) people who have switched to low-tar or to filter cigarettes seem to have, as a consequence, lower lung cancer risks per cigarette (Hammond et al., 1977; Wynder et al., 1976).

Perhaps more surprisingly, lung cancer risks at 60 years of age also depend strongly on the degree of exposure of the lungs to cigarette smoke during the first decade or so of adult life (text-fig. E1). The strength of the dependence (among continuing cigarette smokers) of lung cancer risks in old age on cigarette smoking habits in early adult life means that lung cancer rates among people in their sixties during the 1970's are strongly influenced by the smoking habits in about 1930 of the teenagers and people in their early twenties, a delay of about half a century. It also means that the trends of half a century ago in cigarette usage by young adults will be important determinants of current trends in lung cancer among old people. Analogous large effects of exposure in early "adult" life on cancer risks in later life are also seen in controlled experiments involving the regular application of one of the cancer-causing components of cigarette smoke to laboratory mice (Peto et al., 1975),

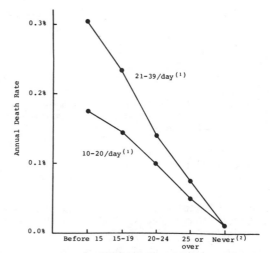

Age (years) when Started to Smoke Cigarettes

TEXT-FIGURE E1.—Data on U.S. veterans (Kahn, 1966). Lung cancer mortality at ages 55–64 among current smokers of cigarettes only, in relation to the age when cigarette smoking first began (though this was perhaps not when regular consumption of substantial numbers of cigarettes first began).

[1] The figures 10–20 and 21–39/day refer to the maximum rate at which the subject ever normally smoked cigarettes; the lifelong average may, of course, be much less than this.

[2] Subject may previously have smoked "once in a while but not every day."

so there is no reason to distrust the importance of early exposure which is apparent in the uncontrolled human data. The human data in text-figure E1 deserve careful examination, because it is impossible to interpret properly the recent lung cancer trends in any developed country unless one appreciates the crucial importance of cigarette smoking in *early* life (as well as the importance of more recent exposure, of course).

Thus lung cancer risks at age 60 years certainly depend very strongly on cigarette usage both at ages 15–25 and at ages over 45. Presumably, they also depend to some extent on cigarette usage at ages 25–45, though the strength of this dependence is not known. Therefore, to interpret in any detail the lung cancer rates among people of a particular age, we ideally need to know not only what they have been smoking in the recent past but also what they smoked decades ago in their teens or twenties. Moreover, to interpret recent lung cancer *trends* among people of a given age, we ideally need to know not only the recent *trends* in adult cigarette consumption but also the *trends* in cigarette consumption by teenagers or young adults in the distant past.

Trends in U.S. Smoking and Lung Cancer

Unfortunately, of course, the exact smoking habits of the young in the distant past are not known. Estimates of varying degrees of reliability have been made, but none can be accepted with confidence, and we prefer to base our inferences chiefly on the total sales of manufactured cigarettes, which should be reasonably reliably known,[1] together with the observation (Surgeon General, 1980) that female cigarette usage seemed to lag about 25 or 30 years behind male cigarette usage.

The major changes in American smoking habits in this century have been the rise in cigarette usage (text-fig. E2) in the first half of the century and the subsequent halving of tar yields per cigarette (Owen, 1976). One cannot, of course, predict from these crude total sales data the exact relative risks of different generations, because neither the ages of the people who smoked the cigarettes sold in past years nor the "style" in which they smoked their cigarettes is known.[2]

---

[1] Questionnaires seeking recall of quantitative smoking habits in the distant past are notoriously unreliable, and even questionnaires about current habits may be subject to large errors. For example, data from four large questionnaire-based surveys (1964, 1966, 1970, 1975) suggest about a 15% reduction between 1964 and 1975 in the number of cigarettes smoked per U.S. adult, but this reduction is probably chiefly due to progressive increases in underreporting (Warner, 1978), because no such large trends are evident in the more reliable data on the numbers of cigarettes actually manufactured. By 1975, 50% more cigarettes were being sold than the questionnaire surveys indicated were being smoked.

[2] The "style" includes stub length, puff frequency, puff size, depth of inhalation, and possibly even speed of inhalation, since this may affect the net exposure of the walls of the large upper airways (which are the part of the lung at greatest risk of cancer) to the carcinogen-carrying droplets or gases in cigarette smoke.

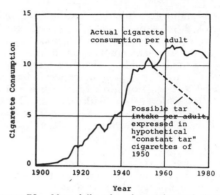

TEXT-FIGURE E2.—Mean daily sales of manufactured cigarettes per U.S. adult over 18 years of age (Surgeon General, 1980), together with a crude estimate of tar yield per adult, based on Owen, 1976. *The estimate of tar yield allows approximately for decreases since 1954 in tar yield per cigarette smoked in a standard manner (but not for any hypothetical compensatory increases in number of puffs per low-nicotine cigarette).*

Moreover, if dietary factors affect lung cancer (*see* section 5.3) these too may change with time. Therefore, there seems little point in trying to devise complex mathematical predictive formulas based on detailed models. Instead, we shall exemplify the qualitative ways in which trends in tobacco exposure might be the chief determinants of the lung cancer trends by a detailed discussion of one particular comparison—that between the lung cancer rates of men aged 45–49 in 1937, 1957, and 1977.

Example: Trends in lung cancer mortality among U.S. males aged 45–49, as we go from 1937, to 1957, to 1977.—Men aged 45–49 in 1937: These men were born in about 1890, and because they grew up before World War I (which ended in 1918) very *few* of them smoked substantial numbers of manufactured cigarettes regularly from early adult life (text-fig. E2). However, *many* will have smoked pipes and/or cigars (which both confer some risk of lung cancer, though not nearly as large a risk as do cigarettes), and a few may have smoked hand-rolled cigarettes.

Men aged 45–49 in 1957: These men were born in about 1910, and because they grew up between the two wars, when the average usage of manufactured cigarettes was 3 or 4/adult/day (text-fig. E2), *some* of them smoked substantial numbers of cigarettes regularly from early adult life, whereas *some* then smoked pipes and/or cigars. However, compared with the cigarettes already being used by young men between the wars, these other forms of tobacco may, by the 1930's, have had a relatively unimportant added effect on the young men's future lung cancer risks. (When a new habit, such as the use of marijuana in recent years, is in the process of being adopted by a country, it tends to be the young adults who adopt it most vigorously.)

Men aged 45–49 in 1977: These men were born in about 1930, and because they grew up after World War II (which ended in 1945), when the average cigarette usage was about 10/adult/day (text-fig. E2), *many* of them smoked substantial numbers of cigarettes regularly from early adult life, while probably by then relatively *few* of them smoked much pipe or cigar tobacco; for the inevitable tendency of the young to be in the forefront of new drug usage seems likely to be accentuated by the disruption of their habits and values that follows a long war with widespread military conscription. (A possible analogy might be with the recent Vietnam War, which may have particularly affected the use of marijuana and other drugs by *young* adults.)

If these three successive generations of men (born 1890, 1910, and 1930) had subsequently all smoked similarly from the age of 25 or 30 onward, one might have expected excess lung cancer risks at ages 45-49 in approximate proportion to the exposure of their lungs to the carcinogenic agents in tobacco smoke in early adult life (text-fig. E1), but, of course, they were not similarly exposed in later life. The men born in 1890 had their "later life" between the wars (when the national average was still only 3 or 4 cigarettes/adult/day plus still some pipe and cigar tobacco), the men born in 1910 had their later life after World War II (when the average was 10 cigarettes/adult/day), and the men born in 1930 had their later life in the 1960's and 1970's [when the average cigarette consumption per adult had not changed much further but the tar yield per cigarette smoked under standard laboratory conditions had decreased by about half (Owen, 1976), which presumably reduces the human tar yield per cigarette by some worthwhile amount (Wald et al., 1980b) and seems to reduce the lung cancer risk per cigarette (Wynder et al., 1976; Hammond et al., 1977)].

From these data on consumption, one might expect approximately a doubling of risk at ages 45-49 between the successive generations born in 1910 and 1930, because *a*) between the times when they were both young adults there was about a threefold increase in cigarette usage per adult with no large change in tar delivery per cigarette, but *b*) between the times when they were both aged about 40 years there was a large decrease (perhaps by about one-third) in the human tar yield per cigarette with no large change in cigarette usage.

The magnitude of the increase in risk between the generations born in 1890 and in 1910 is more difficult to predict because of uncertainty as to how much *young* adults smoked as well as the uncertainty in the relative contributions of pipes, cigars, and cigarettes. If hypothetical effects of hypothetical improvements in nutritional status are ignored, one might approximately expect a fourfold increase due to perhaps a doubling of net exposure of the lungs to carcinogens in early life and perhaps a doubling of net exposure in later life.

Having discussed at length what lung cancer changes we might *expect* to see, we shall now discuss what we *do* see. Among American non-smokers aged 45-49, the annual lung cancer death rate per million men is about 50 (Hammond, 1966). Among all U.S. males aged 45-49, the lung cancer death rates per million were 150 in 1937, 300 in 1957, and 500 in 1977, in round numbers.[3] Therefore, the excess risks ascribable to tobacco were probably about 100, 250 and 450. These figures are reasonably compatible with our crude predictions (of a fourfold increase and then a twofold increase) based on the cigarette consumption data. Note particularly that, comparing 1957 with 1977, the net increase in lung cancer is composed of an increase in young people's smoking long ago, between 1930 and 1950, and a more recent decrease in tar yields, between the 1950's and the 1970's. (Looking further ahead, during the 1980's there should be a worthwhile decrease in the U.S. lung cancer death rates among men aged 45-49. This predicted decrease involves comparison of men born about 1930 with men born about 1940, and the ones born around 1940 should have been exposed to substantially lower net tar deliveries either at ages 15-30, or at ages 30-45, or both.)

Terminology: The "successive generation effect."— Because we were examining a middle-aged group of men (aged 45-49 yr), there was a delay of some 30 years between cause (in the form of trends in teenage cigarette use) and full effect, but if we had been examining older men (e.g., aged 65-69 years), there would have been an even longer delay ($\approx$50 yr) between cause and full effect. These long delays are sometimes described in terms of a "latent period," but this terminology may misleadingly suggest a fixed delay (e.g., of 30 yr) between cause and effect. The reality is more complex, of course, and it is perhaps preferable to speak of a "successive generation effect," whereby the risks among successive generations of men are directly dependent not only on their recent smoking habits (i.e., over the past decade or so) but also on the predisposition to lung cancer which has been imprinted on them by their smoking habits in the distant past. The "successive generation effect" and recent smoking habits *together* determine current lung cancer risks, and neither should be ignored. (For example, if the "successive generation effect" were ignored, one might mistakenly predict a decrease in male lung cancer at ages 45-49 between 1957 and 1977 due to the decrease in tar yields, whereas in fact an increase should be expected.)

Note that although we have emphasized chiefly the importance of cigarette smoking in very early life (i.e., at ages 15-25 or so), in imprinting various different predispositions to subsequent lung cancer on successive generations of men, the amounts smoked at 25-35 (and possibly even at 35-45) must also be of some importance. It is obviously very wrong to ignore exposure

---

[3] The death certification rates were 127, 305, and 497 (table E1 on page 1296), and in table E2 (*see* below) we shall suggest that the 1937 lung cancer death certification rate for people aged 45-49 may have been between 71 and 87% of the true 1937 lung cancer death rate.

in early adult life, but conversely it is an over-simplification to imagine that what happens in the age range 15-25 is the sole determinant of the predispositions that are imprinted on successive generations.

The midcentury peak in tar intake per young male.—Lacking objective data, we shall assume that the net exposure of young men to cigarette smoke during 1900-50 was, very roughly, proportional to the cigarette consumption per adult indicated by the left half of text-figure E2 and that after 1950 it was roughly proportional to the tar yield per adult indicated by the *broken line* in the right half of this graph. There are many possible sources of bias in this approximation,[4] but some may cancel each other out.

Our main conclusion, however, is that among young American men there must have been a fairly sharp peak in net exposure to cigarette smoke around the middle of the century (probably occurring at some time between 1945 and 1955, depending on trends in consumption by the young and on exactly when tar yields first began to drop rapidly) with a substantial decrease thereafter from the mid-century peak values.

Steady increase in tar intake per young female.—The Surgeon General (1980) has suggested that female smoking has lagged about 25 or 30 years behind male cigarette smoking. If the left half of text-figure E2 is shifted to the right by a quarter of a century, it suggests negligible cigarette usage by females in the 1920's, with steady increases thereafter, at least to the mid-1960's. (This is borne out by estimates of the percentages of women who smoked cigarettes, which continue to increase rapidly up to the 1960's.) The tar intake per young female must therefore have risen rapidly up to the 1950's,[5] and although it may have continued to rise thereafter (or may have flattened out thereafter), it can hardly have decreased much, at least during 1955-75. (For example, the proportion of females aged 15-16

---

[4] One large source of bias is that, if they have enough money to indulge their inclinations, young men are more inclined than other adults are to be at the forefront of adoption of a habit such as cigarette smoking while it is spreading, especially in or after prolonged wars. This tendency would increase the consumption per young male in the early years relative to text-fig. E2 (except that America was not very heavily involved in World War I, and that before 1945 the young did not have much spare money). Another large source of bias is that between 1920 and 1970 female smoking has been increasing fairly steadily, which again would increase the consumption per young male in the early years relative to text-fig. E2 and would make the decrease in exposure per young male since 1950 even steeper than it seems in the *broken line* in the text-figure. Finally, changes in the style of smoking (e.g., stub length, puff frequency, puff size, and speed and depth of inhalation) may bias trends in tar exposure among young men quite substantially, but in ways that are impossible to document (except that some compensation for the recent decreases in nicotine and tar seems likely).

[5] The rise will be even larger than might be anticipated just from changes in the composition and numbers of cigarettes that women smoke if American women resemble British women in having also increased the vigor with which they smoke individual cigarettes (Doll et al., 1980).

who smoked cigarettes rose from 10% in 1968 to 20% in 1974: Surgeon General, 1980.)

Decreasing tar intake per mature adult in recent decades.—To make sense of the post-1950 lung cancer trends, we needed some estimate of the tar intake per *young* adult throughout the century (*see* above), together with some estimate of the tar intake per mature adult since World War II ended in 1945. For mature males, tar intake must have been roughly constant for a time and then decreased with decreasing tar levels. For mature females, tar intake must have risen to a maximum at some time between 1945 and 1965 and then likewise decreased.

Male lung cancer data.—From the foregoing crude estimates of trends over previous decades in tar intake by young and by mature males, one might expect lung cancer rates among older males still to be rising, since the increases in smoking by young males before World War II outweigh the decreases in tar yields among mature males in recent decades. Although the generations of men born in 1910, 1920, and 1930 all passed through the sharp "mid-century peak" of tar intake (the generation of 1930 doing so at ages 15-25), the generations born in 1940 and 1950 missed it. Therefore, although one cannot predict from the tobacco data alone whether the male generation of 1920 or the male generation of 1930 will be at greatest risk, the male generations born after 1930 should be at successively lower risk. This is indeed so (table E1, text-fig. E3), and

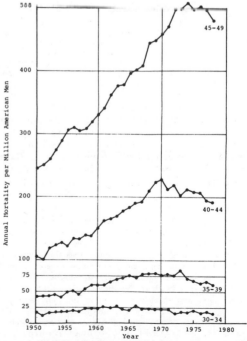

TEXT-FIGURE E3.—Trends since 1950 in lung cancer mortality in U.S. males at young ages; recent decreases are shown for the age groups 30-34, 35-39, 40-44, and 45-49 years.

TABLE E1.—*Annual death certification rates/million people for all races in the United States, from cancer of the lung*[a] The more reliable figures are in boldfaced type.[b,c]

Age, yr	Sex	Annual death certification rates/million people, for:									
		1933–37 (≈1935)[b]	1938–42 (≈1940)[b]	1943–47 (≈1945)[b]	1948–52 (≈1950)[b]	1953–57 (≈1955)	1958–62 (≈1960)	1963–67 (≈1965)	1968–72 (≈1970)	1973–77 (≈1975)	1978 only
30–34	♂	12	15	17	17	**19**	**24**	**24**	**21**	**18**	17
	♀	8	8	8	8	**8**	**8**	**10**	**11**	**10**	11
35–39	♂	26	31	39	44	**46**	**60**	**73**	**78**	**71**	62
	♀	14	13	18	16	**17**	**22**	**28**	**37**	**36**	35
40–44	♂	56	73	94	107	**128**	**151**	**183**	**219**	**206**	192
	♀	25	27	29	29	**34**	**46**	**64**	**87**	**102**	108
45–49	♂	101	153	187	246	**297**	**333**	**392**	**465**	**502**	480
	♀	37	45	52	52	**58**	**79**	**114**	**161**	**212**	235
50–54	♂	159	243	353	467	**578**	**669**	**767**	**871**	**949**	1,021
	♀	56	68	81	81	**84**	**109**	**164**	**269**	**333**	408
55–59	♂	211	347	542	739	**960**	**1,142**	**1,279**	**1,505**	**1,583**	1,647
	♀	84	100	125	116	**116**	**145**	**206**	**349**	**490**	571
60–64	♂	237	408	641	969	**1,320**	**1,665**	**1,975**	**2,247**	**2,486**	2,625
	♀	105	131	159	164	**159**	**184**	**247**	**389**	**617**	767
0–64[d,e]	♂	47	73	105	143	**183**	**219**	**254**	**293**	**314**	325
	♀	19	23	27	27	**27**	**34**	**47**	**73**	**100**	118
65–69[c]	♂	244	417	630	1,052	1,582	2,064	**2,571**	**3,110**	**3,390**	3,557
	♀	124	164	194	218	220	231	**294**	**460**	**671**	876
70–74[c]	♂	235	378	588	1,032	1,551	2,113	**2,740**	**3,551**	**4,186**	4,522
	♀	148	179	239	286	279	282	**332**	**483**	**691**	871
75–79[c]	♂	233	370	530	928	1,355	1,804	**2,572**	**3,453**	**4,358**	4,760
	♀	139	187	255	364	361	344	**372**	**498**	**683**	864
80–84[c]	♂	170	295	421	770	1,148	1,523	**2,046**	**2,913**	**3,814**	4,580
	♀	113	166	215	357	391	394	**411**	**537**	**646**	802
85+[c]	♂	153	223	319	676	876	1,209	**1,574**	**2,173**	**2,754**	3,165
	♀	72	118	161	353	370	402	**451**	**557**	**652**	686
65+[c,d]	♂	224	369	552	963	1,428	1,902	**2,482**	**3,202**	**3,792**	4,136
	♀	128	169	218	290	294	298	**344**	**490**	**675**	850

[a] Estimated as "all respiratory sites except larynx."

[b] Rates in or before 1950 become progressively less reliable the farther back one goes, and are affected by minor errors of population undercount and by the exclusion of cancers of the nose, nasal sinuses, and other sites. (See tables E2 and E3 for corrected estimates.)

[c] Rates at ages >65 yr are progressively less reliable with increasing age.

[d] Standardized to the age distribution of respondents to the U.S. 1970 census (see appendix A).

[e] Standardization to ages 0–64 yr conceals the differences in direction between the recent trends above and below the age of 50 yr.

these decreases should continue through the 1980's (and during the 1980's should spread to the age groups 50–54 and 55–59, of course). Text-figure E3 presents the rates only from 1950 onward, for reasons which have already been discussed at length in appendixes B, C, and D, but some of these reasons probably apply with greater force to lung cancer[6] than to any other

[6] In 1900, most people dying of lung cancer would never have been diagnosed as having lung cancer, either while still alive or (since only a minority of people would have been examined post mortem) after having died of lung cancer. Over the subsequent 50 years the techniques for diagnosing lung cancer were enormously improved by the introduction of X-rays, bronchoscopy, intrathoracic surgery, and sputum cytology, by increasingly reliable distinction between primary and secondary cancer in the lung, and by the introduction of sulfa drugs and antibiotics which cured potentially fatal chest infections due to unrecognized cancers and so permitted those cancers to be recognized. Moreover, medical coverage of the population improved. In 1900 many lung cancer patients would never have been admitted to hospital, but by the middle of the century Americans of working age who developed lung cancer would

typically be investigated in hospital, with postmortem examinations of many who died before a definitive diagnosis had been established. By 1950 most people dying in middle age of lung cancer would probably have been correctly diagnosed, either before or after death, and no great improvements in diagnostic technology for lung cancer have been introduced since then. This improved diagnosis may have been of little value for the patient (since ≈90% of all cases of lung cancer are still incurable when diagnosed), but it improved the accuracy of death certification, producing large artifactual upward trends in lung cancer death certification rates throughout the first half of this century. These artifactual trends were so large in the early period (Enstrom, 1979) that we shall present the data only from 1933, the year in which nationwide collection of causes of death in America began. Even between 1933 and 1950, however, some fairly large artifactual trends must also have occurred, chiefly upward. (As the correct diagnosis of lung cancer became less and less of a medical rarity between 1900 and 1933, an increasing tendency to misdiagnose other causes of death as "cancer of the lung" may have developed, accentuating the artifactual upward trends. Progressive elimination of such errors around the middle of the century may then have diluted slightly the real upward postwar trends. This slight dilution could, of course, be important only where the absolute rates are low and the real upward trends are not large, as, for example, among American females between 1940 and 1960.)

TABLE E2.—*Approximate undercertification factors during 1933–52[a,b,c]*

Age, yr	Estimated undercertification for:			
	1933–37	1938–42	1943–47	1948–52
40–44 (and younger)	0.86	0.93	1.00	1.00
45–49	0.71	0.87	1.00	1.00
50–54	0.69	0.84	1.00	1.00
55–59	0.72	0.86	1.00	1.00
60–64	0.64	0.80	0.97	1.00
65–69	0.57	0.75	0.89	1.00
70–74	0.52	0.63	0.84	1.00

[a] The undercertification factor is here defined as the ratio of the recorded to the true lung cancer death rate. This table lists the undercertification factors indicated in years 1933–37, 1938–42, and 1943–47 if ♀ death certification rates in 1948–52 were about right, and ♀ rates in earlier quinquennia differed from the 1948–52 rates because of undercertification.

[b] What would ideally be required would be separate estimates of the probabilities that ♀ lung cancer will be correctly certified, and that ♀ non-lung cancer will be miscertified as lung cancer. These two ideal probabilities might carry over more accurately to the ♂ data than the above single undercertification factors do.

[c] The contemporary degree of undercertification in England and Wales might be roughly similar, so in correcting British rates for 1941–45 we have used the simple average of these U.S. correction factors for 1938–42 and 1943–47.

TABLE E3.—*Estimated true male U.S. lung cancer death rates in years 1933–52[a]*

Age, yr	Estimated true U.S. mortality rates/ million people, for:			
	1933–37	1938–42	1943–47	1948–52[b]
30–34	14	16	17	17
35–39	30	33	39	44
40–44	65	78	94	107
45–49	142	176	187	246
50–54	230	289	353	467
55–59	293	403	542	739
60–64	370	510	661	969
65–69[c]	428	556	708	1,052
70–74[c]	452	600	700	1,032
75–79[d]	—	—	—	—
80–84[d]	—	—	—	—
85+[d]	—	—	—	—

[a] These are the ♂ mortality rates that would be obtained if the undercertification factors indicated by the ♀ trends during this period (table E2) are applied to the ♂ lung cancer death certification rates/million people.

[b] Actual ♂ rates, because correction factors for 1948–52 are all 1.00.

[c] Less reliable than rates in middle age.

[d] Too unreliable for any useful estimation to be possible.

TABLE E4.—*Mortality in England and Wales from cancer of the lung, estimated as all respiratory, excluding larynx[a,b]*

Age, yr	Sex	Annual death certification rates/million people, for:							
		1942–45[c] (≈1943)	1946–50[c] (≈1948)	1951–55 (≈1953)	1956–60 (≈1958)	1961–65 (≈1963)	1966–70 (≈1968)	1971–75 (≈1973)	1976–79 (1/1/1978)
30–34	♂	39 (40)	41 (41)	38	37	33	25	24	17
	♀	14 (15)	15 (15)	16	15	11	12	9	8
35–39	♂	87 (90)	97 (97)	101	95	92	77	58	56
	♀	25 (26)	27 (27)	30	33	33	32	26	23
40–44	♂	203 (210)	242 (242)	253	256	228	220	177	137
	♀	39 (40)	51 (51)	54	63	71	84	68	62
45–49	♂	404 (432)	555 (555)	589	597	570	537	506	400
	♀	63 (67)	77 (77)	92	108	140	161	183	163
50–54	♂	626 (680)	972 (972)	1,242	1,260	1,234	1,172	1,075	1,019
	♀	102 (111)	123 (123)	144	175	224	290	331	359
55–59	♂	924 (994)	1,375 (1,375)	2,033	2,338	2,299	2,219	2,085	1,891
	♀	135 (145)	176 (176)	214	248	315	409	500	551
60–64	♂	1,073 (1,212)	1,749 (1,776)	2,591	3,347	3,687	3,719	3,561	3,349
	♀	186 (210)	235 (239)	295	342	432	527	678	833
65–69[c]	♂	1,031 (1,257)	1,798 (1,903)	2,964	3,965	4,879	5,304	5,215	4,986
	♀	222 (271)	315 (333)	369	396	532	673	819	992
70–74[c]	♂	799 (1,087)	1,442 (1,567)	2,678	3,924	5,020	6,252	6,899	6,694
	♀	251 (341)	337 (366)	408	470	560	748	900	1,082
75–79[d]	♂	685[e]	1,130[e]	2,087	3,345	4,530	5,931	7,425	8,033
	♀	238[e]	328[e]	436	494	582	741	923	1,117
80–84[d]	♂	—[f]	791[e]	1,444	2,271	3,423	4,578	6,160	7,554
	♀	—[f]	297[e]	402	461	565	661	905	1,008
85+[d]	♂	—[f]	497[e]	927	1,438	2,062	3,490	4,457	5,484
	♀	—[f]	201[e]	316	399	480	629	795	899

[a] Estimates corrected for undercertification (by the same factors as in the U.S. data; *see* table E2) appear in brackets after the data for 1941–45 and 1946–50. The more reliable figures are given in boldface type.

[b] To match the corresponding U.S. data in table E1, cancers of the nose and nasal sinuses start to be included after 1950, at which time they account for only 1% of respiratory cancer deaths.

[c] Moderately unreliable.

[d] Very unreliable, especially in early years.

[e] Correction not attempted for early years; true rates cannot be estimated directly.

[f] Published data not subdivided above 80.

common type of cancer, and some self-explanatory corrected estimates for the male rates in the early years are suggested in tables E2 and E3. Readers who are unhappy with these particular corrections may devise alternative corrections, or they may ignore the data prior to 1950 as being wholly untrustworthy.[7] It would not, however, be advisable to infer from the trends in *uncorrected* lung cancer death *certification* rates before 1950 that any large upward trends in real lung cancer onset rates were taking place among American females or that the trends among males were as steep as the uncorrected data suggest. (Likewise, the trends since 1950 among very old Americans of either sex may be seriously in error.)

Examination of the top right-hand corner of table E1 shows that all the male lung cancer rates above the age of 50 have risen steadily from 1950 to 1978. Probably, however, for the reasons already discussed the rate among men aged 50-54 will reach a maximum by about 1980, the rate among men aged 60-64 will reach a maximum by about 1990 (or a little earlier, especially if tar yields continue to fall), and the rates for men in their 70's will reach a maximum by the turn of the century or earlier, after which male lung cancer rates as a whole should, other things being equal, be decreasing.

Female lung cancer data.—It is not surprising that nearly all the female rates in table E1 are still rising; indeed, it is slightly surprising, and rather encouraging, that the female rates at ages 30-39 seem to have stopped rising recently. A reasonable hope is that in view of the continuing decreases in tar yields, these particular female rates will not start to rise again. However, in view of the increase in female usage of cigarettes right up to the mid-1970's it is too soon to be certain. *If* this halt in the increase of lung cancer mortality for women in their thirties continues, then presumably it will gradually spread to older age groups of women. For example, since there has been no upward trend in lung cancer among women who were in their thirties during the 1970's, there should be no upward trend in lung cancer among these same women as they reach their fifties during the 1990's. This would suggest that by the turn of the century lung cancer rates among middle-aged women will no longer be rising. However, rates among older women will probably (depending on trends in tar yields and female cigarette usage in the intervening period) still be increasing due to the successive increases in tobacco exposure during early adult life of the successive generations of women born in 1920, 1930, and 1940.

Comparison of British and American Trends

Well over 90% of lung cancer deaths occur over the age of 50 where uniform upward trends in U.S. lung cancer mortality have been observed for decades. Yet, our interpretation of current trends in lung cancer mortality and our predictions of future lung cancer mortality depend chiefly on the small decreases that have been observed in recent years in the death rates among men aged under 50. This situation looks a bit like the "tail wagging the dog," and although we intended to avoid theoretical models, there is obviously a sense in which any predictions for 1980-2000+ are theoretical. However, the pattern of rapid increases in all age groups of men for a few decades, followed by gentle decreases first among men in early middle age, then among men in later middle age, and finally by older men, that we have predicted is not only what might theoretically be expected but also, more importantly, what has actually been observed in Britain and Finland, two countries where cigarettes have been used for many decades. It is therefore of interest to compare the American experience to date with the British and Finnish experience.

Cigarette usage by young British men.—Cigarette usage per adult in Britain and the United States is compared in text-figure E4. As has already been noted, the low usage per adult in the early period does not necessarily indicate a correspondingly low intake per young man. In both countries, to estimate the general shape of a graph of cigarette usage per young man in the early period, it *might* be reasonable to take the shapes of the graphs of U.S. and U.K. smoking before 1950 that are suggested by text-figure E4 and roughly double the figures for 1900-20. (World War I, which ended in 1918, would, of course, accentuate the difference in attitudes, values, *and habits* between young and old.) This procedure would suggest that during the 1920's and 1930's the cigarette smoking habits of young men in both countries either increased by a small amount or were approximately constant and that the increase in cigarette usage per adult between the wars was due chiefly to the spread of the habit to middle-aged and older men, and to women. Detailed data for the smoking habits of young men during 1900-40 do not exist in either country,[8] and we justify our rough suggestions partly by their intrinsic plausibility and partly by the unpleasantly circular argument that they do predict something like the observed lung cancer trends.

In Britain, cigarette usage per man has been constant since 1950 (the increases in text-figure E4 being due to

---

[7] Our view is that absolute mortality trends in the early years are difficult to estimate directly, but that trends in the ratio of male-to-female death certification rates at some particular age (e.g., 50-54) are not plausibly accounted for by artifacts of diagnosis, certification, or population estimation and are, therefore, informative. For further discussion of the biases and trends in the pre-1950 lung cancer data, *see* Dorn (1954).

---

[8] Detailed estimates of the exact age-specific cigarette usage by British men have been suggested by the Tobacco Research Council and appear in various of their publications (e.g., Lee, 1976), but these estimates are based on the unsupported assumption that the age distribution of cigarette usage did not change between the 1890's and the 1940's. This assumption does not appear to us to be plausible.

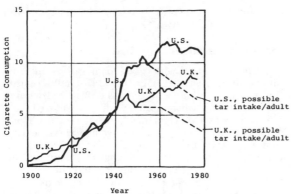

TEXT-FIGURE E4.—Mean daily sales of manufactured cigarettes per U.S. adult over 18 years of age contrasted with the corresponding mean per U.K. adult over 15 years of age (Surgeon General, 1980; Lee, 1976).

Since 1948 there have been annual surveys of British smoking habits (Lee, 1976), and although consumption per woman has risen steadily, consumption per male has remained constant. Broken lines provide a very crude and approximate estimate of tar intake per adult, expressed in "constant tar cigarettes" (Owen, 1976; Wald et al., 1981). British tar yields per cigarette were down 9% by the mid-1950's, down a further 14% by the mid-1960's, and down a further 27% by the mid-1970's; thus tar intake per British male has progressively decreased since 1948.

increases in female smoking), but tar yields per cigarette have been decreasing ever since World War II, so tar intake per young British man may have been roughly constant from the 1920's to 1950, with progressive decreases thereafter—a pattern very different from the sudden American midcentury peak in tar intake. Because of this, the "successive generation effect" (whereby differences between successive generations in smoking in early adult life imprint on those generations differences in predisposition to lung cancer in later life) may have roughly ended in Britain with the generation born early in this century. Consequently, the effects of the large decreases in tar yields per cigarette should be seen more easily in Britain than in the United States, for in Britain they are superimposed for many age groups on a gently rising or roughly constant (we cannot tell which) "successive generation effect"; whereas in the United States they are, initially at least, superimposed on, and therefore concealed by, the large "successive generation effect" increases due to the large mid-century peak in American tar intake, which Britain did not share.

British lung cancer.—The British lung cancer mortality data are conveniently available (Office of Population Censuses and Surveys, 1975) only from 1941 and are presented in table E4. (As with the American data, the British lung cancer data prior to 1950 become progressively less reliable; and the estimates in table E4, which are corrected approximately for under-certification, may be preferred for 1941–45 and 1946–50.) During the 1950's British male lung cancer death rates were decreasing only in the youngest age groups, during the

1960's these decreases had managed to spread throughout middle age (because they did not have to compete with a strong "successive generation effect"), and now they have spread to old age. Among British women, who (like American women) lagged about a quarter of a century behind men in their adoption of cigarettes, the "successive generation effect" is still strong in many age groups, and as yet only below the age of 50 can actual reductions in British female lung cancer rates be seen.

The British and American male mortality data for three particular age groups are contrasted in text-figure E5. Among British men born after the early years of the century, the "successive generation effect" should have moderated, and worthwhile decreases are indeed clearly evident, as should be expected from the postwar decreases in tar yields. (To display rates of 100/million and 5,000/million legibly on one graph, we have used a "log" scale in text-figure E5, on which an increase from 100 to 200 looks as large as an increase from 1,000 to 2,000. This log scale may misleadingly suggest that the decreases are not important, whereas in fact the decrease at ages 40–44 from 256/million to 146/million represents nearly a 50% risk reduction, and even the "slight" decrease at 50–54 represents silent prevention of one-sixth of the lung cancer deaths at these ages.)

The only odd feature of text-figure E5, in view of the similarity of the cigarette sales per adult in Britain and

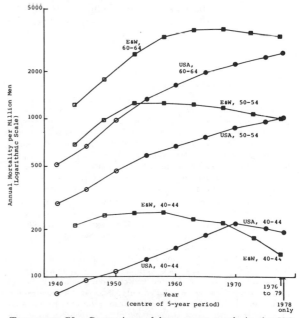

TEXT-FIGURE E5.—Comparison of lung cancer trends in the U.S. (USA, *round symbols*) in selected age groups with corresponding trends in England and Wales (E&W, *square symbols*).
Data from tables E1–E4; points for 1940 to 1950 are estimates corrected for under-certification (open symbols); points for subsequent years are observed rates (solid symbols).

the United States during 1925–40 (text-fig. E4), is that the American death rates for men born in about 1910 are only half the corresponding British rates. It seems probable, however, that the tar intake per young British man between the wars considerably exceeded that per young American man (because of differences in tar intake per cigarette,[9] and possibly also because of differences in the number of cigarettes smoked per young man[10]), and this phenomenon may be the whole explanation for the previous excess British risk. Since 1945, American cigarette usage suddenly began greatly to exceed that in Britain (and the spending power of American youths increased rapidly). Presumably as a result of this, among men aged 40–44 there has been a crossover in about 1970 between British and American lung cancer mortality (text-fig. E5) which is likely to be repeated in about 1980 at ages 50–54 and in about 1990 at ages 60–64. The British data are of interest because, especially in the youngest age groups, they may provide a better indication of the benefits to be expected from changes in cigarette composition, for these benefits are not as completely swamped as they are in most of the American data by the "successive generation effect." Table E5 documents the magnitudes of the risk reductions that have already been observed in England and the United States. Of course, there is no guarantee that cigarette usage has been exactly constant among young adults over the relevant periods, so the true benefits from changes in cigarette composition may be a little less or, more probably, a little more, than is suggested by the comparisons in table E5. However, this table strongly suggests that substantial benefits have already accrued, and it seems

reasonable to expect further substantial decreases during the next decade or two.

Comparison With Finnish Data

Among countries with good data on recent lung cancer and on cigarette usage (Lee, 1975) half a century ago, the only country outside the British Isles and North America where people already smoked substantial numbers of cigarettes between the two World Wars is Finland. In Finland, average cigarette consumption between 1920 and 1940 was 3.7/adult/day, which was then very similar to that in Britain and the United States (text-fig. E4), but Finland, like Britain, did not have the large increase in cigarette usage between 1940 and 1945 that was seen in the United States. Consequently, Finnish lung cancer rates throughout middle age have, like the British rates, already stabilized and begun to fall (table E6).

Table E6 presents lung cancer incidence data and therefore includes both fatal and non-fatal cases. However, if the Finnish rates in the late 1960's are multiplied by about 0.9 to "remove" the non-fatal cases, we get rates in middle age very similar to the corresponding British rates and much higher than the corresponding U.S. rates. Air pollution in rural Finland is negligible (except perhaps in sauna baths!), and even the Finnish cities have never been highly polluted in comparison with British standards. In section 5.7 we did not ascribe any large fraction of lung cancer to air pollution, either acting alone or synergistically with cigarettes. Comparison of the British and Finnish data confirms that *a*) there is no need to assume any large effects of air pollution to get the high levels of lung cancer per cigarette observed in Britain, and that *b*) there is no need to invoke decreases in air pollution to explain the recent decreases in British and American lung cancer mortality.

Other Countries

There are, of course, many countries other than the United States, Britain, and Finland where the relationship between cigarette smoking and lung cancer could have been examined. Although each has its special peculiarities, we know of no country where causes of death are reasonably accurately certified yet the certified lung cancer death rates in middle age are grossly discrepant with what is known of the smoking habits in that country in previous decades. The greatest apparent discrepancy at present is perhaps Japan, where there is less lung cancer than might have been predicted; however, the current rate of increase of Japanese lung cancer death certification rates is so rapid (*see* table 5 on page 1202) that during the 1980's this anomaly may disappear. Because of the strong influence of cigarette consumption in early adult life on lung cancer risks in later life (text-fig. E1), a close correlation between *current* cigarette consumption and *current* lung cancer rates should not exist, especially if

---

[9] In the 1950's, before the advent of filter tips, Americans habitually left much longer "stubs" unburned when they finished each cigarette than did British men (Doll et al., 1959: differences in stub length between American and non-American cigarettes were also obvious to one of us who, in his early teens, habitually scavenged the roads around Southampton docks for smokeable stubs discarded by sailors of various nations). The tar yield from the last few puffs from a short hot stub exceeds that from the first few puffs from a cigarette. In recent decades, however, the advent of filter tips has prevented British men from smoking their cigarettes down to tiny stubs.

[10] *a*) The ratio of young men to adults between the wars was larger in the United States than in Britain, and young men were the principal consumers of cigarettes. The ratio of the number of cigarettes sold to the number of young men would be larger for Britain than for the United States.

b) World War I lasted longer and killed far more young men in Britain than in the United States and so may have produced a larger divergence in attitudes and habits between young and old in Britain. (Although the Vietnam War killed only 1% as large a proportion of young American men as the 1914–18 war killed of British men, it too produced a divergence of attitudes and drug use between young and old.)

c) Any slight differences in average age at starting to smoke substantial numbers of cigarettes regularly could have a large effect on subsequent risks, but there is no evidence bearing on British or American practice on this in earlier decades.

TABLE E5.—*Decreases in lung cancer, comparing 1978 data with data for the worst-affected[a] generations of men in England and Wales and in the United States*

Age, yr	England and Wales				United States			
	Worst-affected[a] generation (born ca. 1910–11)		Rates for 1978 compared with those for worst-affected generation		Worst-affected[a] generation (born ca. 1927–28)		Rates for 1978 compared with those for worst-affected generation	
	Mortality/ million men	Period of observation	Mortality/ million men in 1978	Decrease[b]	Mortality/ million men	Period of observation	Mortality/ million men in 1978	Decrease[b]
30–34	40	1941–45	17	58%/35 yr	24	1958–62	17	30%/18 yr
35–39	98	1946–50	63	36%/30 yr	73	1963–67	62	15%/13 yr
40–44	253	1951–55	138	45%/25 yr	219	1968–72	192	12%/8 yr
45–49	597	1956–60	385	36%/20 yr	502	1973–77	480	4%/3 yr
50–54	1,234[c]	1961–65	1,047	15%/15 yr	?	1980	1,021	—[e]
55–59	2,219[d]	1966–70	1,912	14%/10 yr	?	1985	1,647	—[f]
60–64	3,577[d]	1971–75	3,315	7%/5 yr	?	1990	2,625	—[g]
65–69	5,018[d]	1978	5,018	—	?	1995	3,557	—[g]

[a] These are the generations with the highest death rates at ages 35–44, when substantial effects of smoking first became evident. However, if in the future the number of cigarettes smoked/individual will decrease, or the effective dose of noxious chemicals/cigarette will decrease, the benefits at some particular attained age to these two worst-affected generations may be greater than to the immediately previous generations. The maximum American lung cancer rates in old age may therefore be seen, at around the turn of the century, in the generation born in a few years before this "worst-affected" generation.

[b] Percentage decrease, comparing age-specific mortality in 1978 with that for the worst-affected generation (born 1910–11 in England and Wales, born 1927–28 in United States).

[c] Might have been materially larger but for changes in cigarette composition.

[d] Would have been materially larger but for changes in cigarette composition.

[e] U.S. mortality at ages 50–54 should reach a maximum by ≈1980.

[f] U.S. mortality at ages 55–59 is still rising.

[g] U.S. mortality at ages 60–64 and 65–69 is still rising rapidly.

"current" lung cancer rates are an (age-standardized) average of the lung cancer rates among several different generations of people, each with very different degrees of exposure to cigarette smoke in *early* adult life. If, however, attention is restricted to people of a given age (e.g., 35–44) whose adult lives have been passed under the reasonably stable social conditions that have on the whole prevailed since the end of World War II (and after the end of the immediate postwar austerity period in Europe), there is a reasonable correlation between national cigarette consumption rates per adult when those people were young and their lung cancer risks as they enter middle age (text-fig. E6). This correlation is rather better than we would have expected in view of

the possible international differences in cigarette composition, puff frequency, style of inhalation, butt length, additional use of non-manufactured cigarettes (and other forms of tobacco), and national consumption of cigarettes in the intervening years between 1950 and 1975.[11] However, even if the apparent closeness of the correlation in text-figure E6 is partly due to chance, it does emphasize that the "poor" international correlations that are sometimes used as arguments against the overwhelming importance of tobacco may be "poor" chiefly because they were effectively seeking a correlation between the smoking habits of one generation and the lung cancer risks of their parents or grandparents.

Recapitulation

Current increases in male U.S. lung cancer mortality are following the qualitative pattern that one should expect from the large mid-century peak in cigarette tar intake per U.S. male. Because of this mid-century peak, there have been during recent decades large lung cancer increases due to the "successive generation effect" having imprinted successively increasing predisposi-

TABLE E6.—*Annual lung cancer incidence/million men, Finland[a]*

Age, yr	Annual incidence/million men, for:	
	1967–71	1972–76
30–34	8[b]	11[c]
35–39	56	43
40–44	207	186
45–49	630	518
50–54	1,369	1,340
55–59	2,783	2,514
60–64	4,332	3,923

[a] Average of the 5 most recent available incidence rates (1972–76) and the 5 previous incidence rates (1967–71).

[b] Based on only 6 cases.

[c] Based on only 9 cases.

[11] The effects of the imperfect correlation between the smoking habits of all adults and of young adults in 1950 may be somewhat offset by the presumably opposite effects of this correlation in the intervening years.

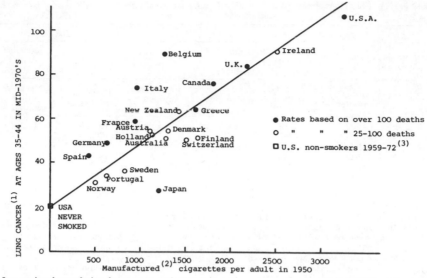

TEXT-FIGURE E6.—International correlation between manufactured cigarette consumption per adult in 1950 while one particular generation was entering adult life (in 1950) and lung cancer rates in that generation as it enters middle age (in the mid-1970's).
Comparison has been restricted to developed countries (i.e., excluding Africa, all of Asia except Japan, and all except North America) with populations >1 million, to improve the accuracy of the observed death certification rates as indicators of the underlying risks of lung cancer among people aged 35–44.

[1] *Lung cancer death certification rates per million adults aged 35–44 are from WHO (1977, 1980). These rates are the means of the male and female rates for all years (1973, 1974, or 1975) reported in WHO (1977), except for Greece [which was not reported in WHO (1977) and thus was taken from WHO (1980)] and Norway, for which the rates in WHO (1977) and WHO (1980) were based on only 11 and 14 cases, respectively; for statistical stability, these were averaged.*

[2] *Manufactured cigarettes per adult are from Lee (1975) for the year 1950 (except for Italy, where consumption data are available in 5-yr groups only; to avoid the temporary postwar shortages, data for 1951–55 have been used). This excludes handrolled cigarettes, which in most countries accounted for only a small fraction of all cigarette tobacco in 1950.*

[3] *U.S. non-smoker rates were estimated by fitting straight lines (on a double logarithmic scale) to the relationships between lung cancer mortality and age reported for male and for female lifelong non-smokers by Garfinkel (1980) and averaging the predicted values at age 40. [Although the average of the male and female rates actually observed at these ages is similar to this estimated value, these observed rates are each based on fewer than 5 cases (Garfinkel, 1980) and so might have been inaccurate.]*

tions to subsequent lung cancer on the successive generations of American men born up to 1930. These increases in lung cancer mortality will probably continue at least up to the turn of the century among older American males.

Quantitatively, the American increases are not quite as large as comparison with Britain and Finland would have led one to expect, possibly because of some relatively less noxious aspect of American cigarette composition and probably because Americans took fewer puffs from each cigarette or in some other way exposed the key target areas in the lungs to less chemical damage per cigarette.

Worthwhile decreases, probably due to the switch to less hazardous cigarettes, are evident in those U.S. age groups (born since 1930) in which the rapid increases due to the "successive generation effect" have abated. Although worthwhile risk reductions may also have been conferred on older age groups by the switch to less hazardous cigarettes, these are not sufficient to override the rapid upward trends still occurring in older age groups due to the "successive generation effect."

In lung cancer, as for most other types of cancer, the key piece of evidence that should be examined to determine the net effects on adults of any new factors that have recently begun to operate is the trend among the *youngest* age groups (e.g., 35–44) in which any material effects of the causative agent could be expected (*see* table D6 on page 1287). If the trend in these *youngest* age groups is downward, as for stomach cancer, female genital cancer, male lung cancer, and pancreatic cancer, any recent net changes are likely to have been for the better, and the effects of these changes will probably spread to older age groups in the future. If the trend in these *youngest* age groups is upward (as for melanoma among males), then the opposite is true. The trends in the older age groups (e.g., 65–74) may chiefly reflect, via the "successive generation effect," the delayed effects of changes in exposure that occurred many decades ago. Consequently, in the trends among older people, the effects of even quite large recent changes in exposure may be difficult to discern (even though complete cessation of smoking leads to very substantial avoidance of risk within less than a decade).

Comparison With Other Interpretations of Trends in U.S. Lung Cancer

The interpretation that we have offered of the U.S. lung cancer trends differs sharply from that put forward by the Council on Environmental Quality in the 1980 inter-agency report to the President of the United States by the Toxic Substances Strategy Committee (entitled "Toxic Chemicals and Public Protection"). The TSSC report, which closely followed an unpublished analysis by Schneiderman (1979), obtained considerable publicity when it was released, both in the lay and scientific press [e.g., the long report in the influential journal *Science* (*209*:998–1002) entitled "Government says cancer rate is increasing"]. The TSSC concluded that large increases in lung cancer were occurring over and above those attributable to smoking, but their analysis was based on the absurd assumption that if American smoking habits (and any other relevant exposures) had been constant from the 1960's to the 1970's there would have been no large trends in lung cancer over this period! This extraordinary failure to expect any large increases due to the "successive generation effect" is a simple scientific error to be corrected, rather than a new scientific hypothesis to be considered, because massive "successive generation effects" have been seen or are being seen in every country that has adopted cigarette smoking on a large scale before the middle of this century. If *new* (e.g., since 1950) toxic chemicals or occupational carcinogens were now having any really substantial effects on U.S. lung cancer trends, then their percentage effect would be expected to be largest among men in their 30's, 40's, and perhaps 50's rather than among men in their 60's and 70's, whereas in fact we observe rapid increases among men in their 70's and *decreases* among men under 50.

Any analysis is bound to be misleading if, as the TSSC did in its Council on Environmental Quality report, it averages together (by age standardization) the upward trends in old age due to the pre-1945 increases in cigarette usage by young adults and the downward trends in early middle age where the pre-1945 increases have had their full effect and so have ceased to dominate the trends. The essence of any reliable interpretation of trends in cancer incidence is separate examination of the trends among each separate age group, as was already being undertaken for U.S. lung cancer mortality more than a quarter of a century ago by Dorn (1954), with conclusions rather similar to our own. Only if no important differences in (at least the directions of) these separate trends is evident should they be averaged together by "age standardization," and even then it is wise not to combine the data for people over 65 with that for people under 65.

Failure to comply with this basic principle of cancer epidemiology (together with various other serious errors of judgment in matters of epidemiology[12] has led the Toxic Substances Strategy Committee to suggest that a large group of cancers are increasing extremely rapidly due to presumably occupational factors. Had they

examined, in a standard way, trends in *mortality* data in middle age or among people aged 35–44 (*see* appendix D), no such conclusion would have emerged.

However, this very fact emphasizes the weakness of any analysis of national trends as a means for detecting the effects of causes of cancer like asbestos which, though important, probably only increase the incidence of some common type of cancer by a few percent (*see* section 5.6). We have scrutinized the U.S. lung cancer trends spanning the postwar period, during which period occupational exposure to asbestos has increased substantially, probably by now causing some thousands of lung cancer deaths a year. However (like the avoidance of some risk in the older age groups due to lowered tar yields), this is not clearly evident from the trends alone. Moreover, it might not have been unequivocally evident even if the large increases due to cigarettes had roughly stabilized long ago. Clearly, the effects of some other cause of cancer as important as asbestos could also lie unnoticed in these trends, especially if, like asbestos, its effect is to multiply up the effects of tobacco.

We have shown that the most important parts of the pattern of trends in age-specific lung cancer death certification rates *can* be explained by plausible assumptions about the effects of smoking, but this does not mean that those plausible assumptions are exactly true. Thus we do not claim to have shown that no important causes lie buried in the lung cancer trends, but merely to have shown that the trends themselves do not provide any strong evidence for the existence of any such causes. Despite this reservation, however, the downward lung cancer trends among males in early adult life remain moderately reassuring.

Trends in Lung Cancer Among U.S. Non-Smokers

This conclusion might in principle be tested in another way by examination of the trend in non-smokers. Enstrom (1979a) has shown that, from 1900 to the present, lung cancer death *certification* rates among non-smokers have risen, the largest relative increase being between 1900 and 1950, which he (and we) dismiss as being largely or wholly an artifact of death certification practice, with both "largely" and "wholly" being possible, and little chance of rendering either implausible. Since 1950 there have also been artifactual

---

[12] The most important other error (apart from implicitly assuming that no "successive generation effects" should exist) was to use, instead of mortality data, the trends in incidence suggested by comparison of the 1969–71 TNCS incidence data with the 1973–76 SEER incidence data. (*See* appendix C for criticism of this procedure.) Lesser errors include the use of "all-ages" rates instead of "under 65" rates (or, preferably, age-specific rates for some middle-aged age groups) and the construction of a category of cancers that were supposed to be those "most likely" to be related to occupational factors, but that included tumor types, such as kidney, melanoma, and myeloma, for which there is little independent evidence to suggest any unusually close relation to occupational factors.

increases in lung cancer death certification rates in old age, but the question that we want to address now is whether since 1950 there has been any material upward trend in the *real* lung cancer death rate among middle-aged non-smokers.[13]

Enstrom (1979a) tried to answer this question in two ways, but both may be seriously biased by confusion of ex-smokers with lifelong non-smokers. In his first method, the numbers of non-smokers in a sample of the U.S. population were estimated directly by questioning the people concerned, so those who described themselves as lifelong non-smokers presumably were. In contrast, to estimate the annual numbers of deaths among lifelong non-smokers, he used data from the national mortality surveys of 1958/59 and 1966/68, in which the smoking habits of some thousands of people who had died of lung cancer were estimated by writing to the "informant" listed on the death certificate (i.e., the person who had informed the U.S. Government of the fact of death) asking various questions about the dead person, one question being whether the dead person had smoked. This method inevitably leads to misclassification of some ex-smokers as being "lifelong non-smokers," and so inevitably leads to an overestimation of the number of lung cancer deaths among "lifelong non-smokers." The magnitude of this overestimation will presumably increase as the lung cancer epidemic increases among smokers. Some estimate of its magnitude in the mid-1960's may be obtained by comparing lung cancer death rates in the American Cancer Society's prospective study of *self*-described non-smokers (Garfinkel, 1980) during 1960–72 with the rates estimated as above from the 1966/68 national mortality survey. Standardized for age,[14] the annual male death rate was 14±1 per 100,000 *self*-described non-smokers versus 25 per 100,000 estimated as described above. This difference suggests that a) the percentage of lung cancer patients who have never smoked may be substantially smaller than is suggested by the national mortality surveys, and b) trends in lung cancer mortality suggested by comparison of these surveys cannot be trusted, especially since the proportion of relatively recent ex-smokers may have altered substantially over the past quarter century, and since the question asked of the informants in the two surveys defined "non-smokers" differently.

---

[13] One might expect such a trend merely from the effects of "passive" smoking on non-smokers (Hirayama, 1981; Trichopoulos et al., 1981), although a) the use of pipes and cigars which preceded use of cigarettes must have created some effects of passive smoking early this century, and b) any effect might take about 20 yr longer than the effects on smokers to show up, since presumably if any material effect of passive smoking really exists then heavy exposure in childhood will ultimately lead to the greatest risk. Also, to judge by the sales of manufactured cigarettes (text-fig. E1), children have been really heavily exposed only since 1945.

[14] Standardized in 10-yr age groups to the population of respondents aged 35–84 to the 1970 U.S. census, taking death rates at ages 75 and over to apply to 75–84.

Enstrom's (1979a) second argument involves the lung cancer death rates observed during the first few years of the two largest American prospective studies of mortality among people who at the beginning of those studies (in the 1950's) said that they had never smoked regularly. These non-smoker lung cancer death rates, relating to about 1960, are then compared with the lung cancer death rates estimated (with some methodological difficulties) during 1968–75 among active Mormons, almost none of whom are current smokers. However, about one-third of active Mormons in California are ex-smokers (Enstrom, 1975, 1978), so although the lung cancer death rates of active Mormons in California and Utah in about 1972 were estimated to be about double those of the self-described *lifelong* non-smokers in about 1960, this is not evidence that non-smoker death rates increased at all between 1960 and the early 1970's.

A more natural comparison would be of the lung cancer death rates among the self-described non-smokers in the early years of these two prospective studies of self-described non-smokers with their death rates in the later years of those same studies, preferably excluding (or examining separately) the first year or two after recruitment because there may well be a shortage of lung cancer deaths in the first year if people who already have lung cancer are not enrolled.

First, in the ACS study, Hammond (1977) determined the smoking habits of one million men and women in 1959 and monitored all causes of death among most of them until mid-1972. Some of the men and many of the women claimed that they had never smoked regularly, and 189 male and 503 female lung cancer deaths accumulated during 1960–1972 among these 1,959 non-smokers (Garfinkel, 1980), but no material trend in lung cancer mortality among middle-aged non-smokers of either sex was evident (Garfinkel L: Personal communication; *see* also Garfinkel L, 1981), a conclusion likely to be strengthened rather than weakened if the first year after recruitment (mid-1960 to mid-1961) were excluded.

Second, Dorn determined the smoking habits of more than a quarter of a million U.S. veterans in 1954 or 1957, and any deaths among them before mid-1970 have been traced (Rogot and Murray, 1980). Detailed data for the non-smokers among these veterans have been made available to us by E. Rogot of the National Heart, Lung, and Blood Institute, and again no evidence of any upward trend in lung cancer among non-smokers is apparent (table E7). Pending further data, we remain unconvinced that any material trends in true lung cancer death rates among American non-smokers have occurred in recent decades (although some such increases should be expected if the effects of "passive" smoking reported by Hirayama (1981) and Trichopoulos et al. (1981) are confirmed). A fortiori, we are even less convinced that any such trends not attributable to passive smoking among non-smokers have occurred. We note that two incidental by-products of the large case-control study of lung cancer in

TABLE E7.—*Lack of apparent upward trend in cancer of the lung, and in other smoking-related types of cancer, among male U.S. non-smokers*[a,b]

Type of cancer	Years since entry to study						
	1	2, 3, 4	5, 6, 7	8, 9, 10	11, 12, 13	14, 15, 16	All study years
Lung, observed	6	24	31	40	41	35	177
Lung, expected[c]	6.5	23.6	30.9	39.2	43.9	33.0	177.0
Ratio:observed/expected	0.9	1.0	1.0	1.0	0.9	1.1	1
Other smoking-related cancers							
MEPL,[d] observed	4	9	9	11	10	6	49
MEPL,[d] expected	2.3	7.4	8.9	10.3	11.6	8.6	49.0
Bladder, observed	9	16	22	17	31	29	124
Bladder, expected	4.0	12.3	16.9	24.4	33.6	32.9	124.0
Pancreas, observed	8	30	42	31	50	34	195
Pancreas, expected	7.9	28.7	36.4	40.5	43.6	37.9	195.0
Total,[e] all above smoking-related cancers							
Total, observed	27	79	104	99	132	104	545
Total, expected	20.6	72.0	93.2	114.3	132.6	112.4	545.0
Ratio:observed/expected	1.3	1.1	1.1	0.9	1.0	0.9	1

[a] Mortality among the 2 samples of male U.S. veterans who, in early 1954 (sample 1) or early 1957 (sample 2), had "never smoked regularly," monitored from mid-1954/57 to mid-1970.

[b] We are greatly indebted to Dr. Eugene Rogot, of the National Heart, Lung, and Blood Institute, who devised and performed these analyses and provided us with the results of them.

[c] Numbers of deaths observed are compared with the (indirectly standardized) numbers expected if, among men of a given single year of age in a given sample, death rates were unrelated to calendar year.

[d] MEPL denotes mouth, esophagus, pharynx, and larynx.

[e] Total of all the above smoking-related cancers (lung, mouth, esophagus, pharynx, larynx, bladder, and pancreas).

relation to smoking habits and occupational factors which we have recommended (in sections 5.1, 5.6, and elsewhere) will be *a*) to provide a direct estimate of the effects on non-smokers of passive smoking by their parents or spouses, and *b*) to provide a direct estimate of the absolute lung cancer death rate among non-smokers, for comparison with the past rates recorded in the above two studies and with any future estimates that may become available later this century.

APPENDIX F: EXAMINATION OF THE ARGUMENTS AND CONCLUSIONS IN "ESTIMATES OF THE FRACTION OF CANCER IN THE UNITED STATES RELATED TO OCCUPATIONAL FACTORS" (OSHA, SEPT. 15, 1978)

In the main text (pages 1240–1241), we stated our opinion that the estimates made in the OSHA document could not be regarded as having any validity, primarily because the implicit assumption was made that the industrial conditions that had been recognized as giving rise to gross hazards of occupational cancer were typical of the conditions to which 11.9 million workers in the United States were currently exposed. We examine here in detail the reasons for our conclusion.

For example, a total of 7,300 excess respiratory cancers (other than nasal sinus cancer) was "projected" (OSHA, 1978) to occur each year in workers exposed to nickel as follows:

A Norwegian study of Pedersen et al. in 1973 observed an overall excess respiratory cancer incidence of 5.6-fold

among nearly 2,000 men exposed to nickel. The highest risk (risk ratio of 14.0) was observed in men first employed before 1930 and followed for at least 40 years. Assessing that an overall risk ratio of about 5 for all respiratory cancers can be applied to the approximately 1,400,000 [U.S.] workers estimated to be exposed to nickel [in 1972], it is projected that about 7,300 excess respiratory cancers, excluding nasal cancer, will occur each year.

Arithmetically, this calculation is correct: The age-adjusted annual risk of lung cancer among males more than 20 years old in the United States was 0.00131, so a fivefold risk ratio would correspond to an excess annual risk of $(5-1) \times 0.00131$, or 0.00524, the multiplication of which by 1.4 million does indeed yield a figure of 7,300. This calculation, however, might fairly be described as a confidence trick. It takes an estimate of risk from Norway and assumes that the same *relative* risk of respiratory cancer would apply to the United States where the normal incidence of the disease was much higher. It further assumes that the 1,400,000 workers currently "exposed to nickel" in the United States have been exposed to the same amounts as men employed in a nickel refinery, most of whom began employment under very dusty conditions [as is made clear in the publication by Pedersen et al. (1973)], despite the fact that many less than 1% of all American nickel workers are employed in refineries, that no hazard from exposure to nickel has been demonstrated outside a refinery, and that it is uncertain which specific nickel compound is carcinogenic to humans (IARC Working Group, 1980). This projected number of incident cases is then approximately doubled,[1] to yield an estimate of about 15,000 lung cancer deaths per year over the next few decades due to exposure to nickel in or before 1972–74.

The impropriety of the whole calculation is underlined by the fact that the risk of respiratory cancer that used to be observed in nickel refineries included a risk of nasal sinus cancer that caused about a third as many excess deaths being certified as being due to cancer of this type as were certified as being due to cancer of the lung, so that the above 15,000 lung cancers suggest that nickel should be responsible over the next few decades for about 5,000 nasal sinus cancer death certificates a year (unless, with the increase in national lung cancer death rates, the ratio of nasal sinus to lung cancer among nickel refiners has greatly decreased). Nickel has been widely used for decades, so if such a total is ever to be attained we should already be a fair way toward it. In fact, in the entire United States during 1973–77 there were on the average only 274 male deaths each year certified as being due to nasal sinus cancer, and it is unlikely that more than about half of these are due to all occupational causes of nasal sinus cancer put together, as an average of 158 such deaths also occurred each year in women. Moreover, no epidemic increases seem likely this century as even these small numbers are decreasing with the passage of time in both sexes. Nasal sinus cancers were not considered in the OSHA report. Had they been, the paradox of predicting that occupational exposure to nickel would cause more than ten times as many deaths to be attributed to nasal sinus cancer as could possibly be the case might have alerted the authors to the unsoundness of their methodology.

The argument that led to the projection of a further 7,300 excess lung cancers each year from current (1972–74) occupational exposure to inorganic arsenic (and therefore again to some 15,000 fatal lung cancers per year from ever-exposure to this agent) was along similar lines. To avoid any risk of misrepresentation, it too is reproduced verbatim from OSHA (1978):

> In 1969 Lee and Fraumeni evaluated the mortality experience of 8,047 white male smelter workers exposed to arsenic trioxide during 1938 to 1963. Smelter workers were found to have a three-fold excess in mortality from all respiratory cancer compared to a statewide population control group. About half of those in the study population were exposed to arsenic less than 10 years. Of those exposed for at least 15 years and followed another 25 years, the relative risk for respiratory cancer was 4.7. If this excess can be applied to the approximately 1,500,000 workers exposed to arsenic, it is projected that about 7,300 excess lung cancers each year may occur.

---

[1] The projected total of 33,000 incident cases of cancer per year ascribed to *current* (1972–74) exposure to nickel, arsenic, chromium, benzene, or other petrochemicals is assumed in the OSHA paper to correspond to 10–20% of 400,000–450,000 cancer deaths per year (i.e., about 64,000 deaths/yr) due to *ever*-exposure to those five agents. *See* section 5.6 for a more detailed description of this aspect of the arguments in the OSHA paper.

Similar risks have been reported for several other groups of copper smelters and for men engaged in the manufacture of pesticides in the United States and elsewhere, all of whom had been heavily exposed to inorganic arsenic in the course of their work. Only one study provides any basis for deriving a relationship between dose and effect and that on a most tenuous basis (Pinto et al., 1977). The World Health Organization (1980) recently used the results of this study to deduce that exposure to 25 μg of inorganic arsenic/m^3 of air at work for 25 years would double the normal risk of lung cancer, but this must be regarded as an overestimate of the effect because the measurements of pollution were made in 1973 at a time when, according to the authors, exposure had already been substantially reduced. Even without this qualification, however, it follows that the population of workers that was studied epidemiologically must have been regularly exposed to concentrations of the order of 100 μg/m^3, and it is impossible to believe that the 1.5 million workers who were said to be "currently exposed" to arsenic could be exposed to anything like that amount. These workers included electroplaters, farmers, jewelers, and plumbers in a list of 78 occupations with potential arsenic exposure published by the Department of Health, Education, and Welfare and include many who are exposed only to organic arsenicals, which have never been shown to cause cancer at all. The Occupational Safety and Health Administration (1976) had, in fact, already lowered its estimate of men and women potentially exposed to inorganic arsenic to about 900,000 of whom "a large number . . . work in areas where exposure to inorganic arsenicals are very low or non-existent," and added that estimates of the number of directly exposed workers at any one time currently ranges from 1,500 to 1,700 for exposure levels of 100 μg/m^3 and above to 7,000 for exposure levels of 4 μg/m^3 and above. Using these dose estimates, one might finish up with an estimate rather similar to that of the American Industrial Health Council (1978), an organ of the chemical industry, which estimated that the maximum number of lung cancers induced by occupational exposure to arsenic that would occur over the next quarter of a century would be 15 a year: that is, about 0.2% of the figure of 7,300 ascribed to recent exposure (or 0.1% of the 15,000 or so ascribed to ever-exposure) in the statement filed at OSHA. In World War II it was possible to arrive at almost exactly the correct number of planes lost by enemy action on either side by calculating the geometric mean of the figures claimed by the British and German authorities. A similar technique would lead to an estimate of 331 lung cancer deaths from occupational exposure to arsenic each year. On the available evidence, however, this figure seems rather high.

For asbestos the authors used two assumptions: *a)* that 4 million American workers have had "heavy exposure to asbestos" since the beginning of World War II and that the proportion who have died or will die of lung cancer, pleural or peritoneal mesothelioma, or gastrointestinal cancer is indicated by Selikoff's studies of various groups of insulation workers and adds up "to a total of 35-44%," as against a proportion of 8-9% who would have been expected to die of cancer of these sites in the absence of exposure to asbestos; and b) that a further 4-7 million workers who have been less heavily exposed experience an excess risk of "one-quarter of that to the heavily exposed workers." It is then deduced from the first assumption that "at least 1.6 million" of the heavily exposed workers "are thus expected to die of the asbestos-related cancers listed above" and from the two assumptions (OSHA, 1978) combined that

> ... the total number of cancers attributable to asbestos in the less heavily exposed group would be expected to be in the range of 0.4 to 0.7 million, raising the total to 2.0 to 2.3 million. Since most of these cancers will be manifested over a period of 30-35 years, the expected average number of cancer deaths associated with asbestos per year in that period will be between 58,000 to 75,000. Such numbers would comprise 13-18% of all cancer deaths expected in the United States in the for[e]seeable future (assuming that total cancer deaths increase to 400,000 to 450,000 per year).

Their argument is impossible to follow in detail, because of the inconsistencies in the allowance that is made for the normal background incidence of cancers of the lung and gastrointestinal tract,[2] the terms "asbestos related," "attributable to asbestos," and "associated with asbestos" being inappropriately interchanged in places. Rectification of these inconsistencies would, however, alter the predictions of the total effects of asbestos by only about one-fifth, which is relatively unimportant. The more important question is whether the large estimates of risk, which the OSHA paper carries over from Selikoff's studies of people who have been occupationally exposed as shipyard insulation workers for decades, really are applicable to about 10% of the men in the whole United States[3] (half of whom are less than 40 years of age). We have no means of testing this directly, but the internal evidence of Selikoff's own studies makes it extremely unlikely. We

note, for example, that the estimate of 8-11 million American workers who had been exposed to asbestos in the United States since the beginning of World War II included 4.5 million who had worked in shipyards during the 1940's and that this work force was extremely mobile with a labor turnover each year that averaged more than 100/100 employees between 1941 and 1945 (Selikoff et al., 1979). The average duration of exposure per man in such a transient work force would, of course, be fairly brief, and of course while they were employed not all of them would be heavily involved with asbestos insulation. In contrast to this, the men that had been studied by Selikoff (42% of the recent deaths among whom were attributed to asbestos-related cancers) were men employed as shipyard insulation workers in 1967 and whose first employment as such had been 20 years or more previously (Selikoff et al., 1979). These were, therefore, for the most part long-term employees with a prolonged and specific exposure to the hazards of insulation, quite different from short-term employees in other shipyard trades.

Another check on the validity of the estimates can be obtained by comparing the estimated numbers of mesothelioma deaths with the numbers that actually occur. Since the authors' figures require 7-10% of heavily exposed workers to die of pleural or peritoneal mesothelioma, it follows from their argument that there should be between 350,000 and 575,000 deaths from asbestos-related mesothelioma over the postulated period of 30-35 years (7-10% of 4 million and one-quarter of 7-10% of 4-7 million; here, the authors' arithmetic inconsistencies in allowing for normal background have a negligible effect, because the spontaneous incidence of mesotheliomas is so small). The claim that these calculations refer mainly to future effects and that "an estimate of the present-day numbers of cancers attributable to asbestos would undoubtedly be smaller" does not make much sense, as the large proportion of asbestos-exposed workers whose exposure was in the shipyards during the war (41-56% of the total) must already be suffering near peak absolute rates, if indeed their peak is not already past due to the normal attenuation of the number at risk through death in old age and the specific attenuation of cigarette smokers due to the multiplicative effect of exposure to the two agents.

If, therefore, the OSHA calculations are correct, and 350,000-575,000 mesotheliomas will really occur over 30-35 years, at least 10,000 per year should be occurring already, and they are not.

Cancer registry data suggest that approximately 900 cases were diagnosed each year in the early 1970's (Hinds, 1978), giving an annual incidence of approximately 7 per million in men and 2 per million in women. A detailed study of 188 cases diagnosed in Los Angeles county between 1972 and 1979, where the incidence in each sex was close to the estimated national rate, suggests that about 70-80% of the male patients and 10-20% of the female patients had been specifically exposed to asbestos (Henderson and Peto,

---

[2] There appear to be two inconsistencies. a) If, as is assumed, 35-44% of heavily exposed men and 8-9% of unexposed men get certain types of cancer, and if, as is assumed, the excess risk among the less heavily exposed is one-quarter that among the more heavily exposed, then it should be 7-9%, not 10%, among the 4-7 million less heavily exposed. b) It is not stated in unequivocal terminology exactly what the figures 2.0 to 2.3 million are supposed to be. If, as the context in subsequent pages makes probable, they refer to the number of deaths that could have been prevented by avoidance of asbestos, then it was an oversight not to have subtracted the 0.35 million background cancers expected anyway among the heavily exposed workers.

[3] OSHA (1978) estimated that approximately 1 million of the 8-11 million American workers who had been exposed to asbestos in the United States since the beginning of World War II had already died, leaving 7-10 million (most of whom would have been male) still alive, which amounts to about 10% of the 1978 U.S. adult male population of 73 million (table B1).

1981). If these results are applicable nationally (and the similarity of the incidence rates suggests that they are), it follows that some 500–600 mesotheliomas were caused by asbestos each year between 1970 and 1975.

Even though mesotheliomas are probably underdiagnosed, and even though the incidence of mesotheliomas among men is increasing, it seems most unlikely that as many as 1,000 per year could be currently caused by asbestos.[4] In other words, there is at least a tenfold exaggeration in the OSHA estimates of the numbers of mesotheliomas due to asbestos and, consequently, in their estimates of the other cancer hazards of asbestos.[5] Errors by at least a factor of 10 were also present in the OSHA estimates of the effects of arsenic and nickel, and no reasons are given for supposing that the errors in their treatment of chromium, benzene, or other petrochemicals were any less extreme.

---

[4] That some mesotheliomas are miscertified as other types of cancer [68% in Selikoff and Seidman's (1980) detailed study] is evident. It is notable, however, that in the recent study of mesotheliomas in residents of a coastal town in Virginia where there were several large shipyards (Tagnon et al., 1980), the incidence of mesothelioma determined from discharge diagnoses, pathology files, tumor registries, and the records of local physicians was not elevated above the nationally recorded rate (Hinds, 1978) for black males and black and white females and was increased only four times for white males among whom (to judge by the control group) 28% at the ages studied had been employed in shipbuilding. It is, therefore, probably generous to double the national figure.

These straightforward arguments are not accepted by people who wish to emphasize the importance of occupational factors (e.g., the Toxic Substances Strategy Committee in its 1980 report to the U.S. President, or Epstein, 1981a, 1981b), although it would be more accurate to say that these arguments are not addressed by such people. The arguments have, however, been discussed with many epidemiologists and have been accepted by most. They are reinforced, as far as asbestos is concerned, by the experience of chest physicians whose clinical practice demonstrates the falsity of the proposition that half their patients with respiratory cancer have had occupational exposure to significant amounts of asbestos which, in three-quarters, could be described as heavy.

REFERENCES

See pages 1260–1265.

---

[5] At the 1981 Cold Spring Harbor Laboratory meeting on the Quantification of Occupational Cancer, the speakers in the session devoted to asbestos came from a range of backgrounds (including Dr. Selikoff's department at New York, the National Cancer Institute, and various industries and universities). Using some quite different epidemiological approaches, several of these speakers devised numerical estimates of the proportion of U.S. cancer deaths currently due to asbestos, all of which were around 1 or 2% (rather than 13–18%!), and no speaker or participant dissented from this consensus.

INDEX